University College Worcester
Library
Henwick Grove, WORCESTER,

The Peirson Library
UNIVERSITY COLLEGE WOI
Henwick Grove, Worcester, \
Tele

A1028798

DISABLED PEOPLE AND EMPLOYMENT

To all the visually impaired physiotherapists who took part in this study

Disabled People and Employment

A study of the working lives of visually impaired physiotherapists

SALLY FRENCH
Senior Lecturer, Department of Management and Social Sciences, King Alfred's College of Higher Education, Winchester, UK

Ashgate

Aldershot • Burlington USA • Singapore • Sydney

© Sally French 2001

All rights reserved. No part of this publication may be reproduced, stored in a retrieval system or transmitted in any form or by any means, electronic, mechanical, photocopying, recording or otherwise without the prior permission of the publisher.

Published by
Ashgate Publishing Limited
Gower House
Croft Road
Aldershot
Hants GU11 3HR
England

Ashgate Publishing Company
131 Main Street
Burlington, VT 05401–5600 USA

Ashgate website: http://www.ashgate.com

British Library Cataloguing in Publication Data
French, Sally
 Disabled people and employment : a study of the working
 lives of visually impaired physiotherapists
 1. Physical therapists 2. Visually handicapped – Employment
 I. Title
 331.5′91

Library of Congress Control Number: 2001091919

ISBN 0 7546 1468 9

Printed and bound in Great Britain by
Antony Rowe Ltd, Chippenham, Wilts.

Contents

List of Figures — vi
List of Tables — vii
List of Abbreviations — ix
Introduction — xi

Part 1 Disabled People and Employment: Theoretical Issues

1. Models of Disability — 3
2. Disability and Employment — 17
3. Disabled Health and Welfare Professionals — 37

Part 2 The Experiences of Visually Impaired Physiotherapists

4. Visually Impaired Physiotherapists: An Historical Overview — 53
5. A Comparison of Visually Impaired and Sighted Physiotherapists — 67
6. Educational Inclusion: Barriers and Coping Strategies — 93
7. Employment: Barriers and Coping Strategies — 117
8. The Changing Work Environment: Its Impact on Visually Impaired Physiotherapists — 145
9. Personal Narratives: Disabling Barriers – Enabling Contexts — 157

Part 3 Overview and Concluding Comments

10. Discussion and Conclusion — 169

Bibliography — 181
Index — 193

List of Figures

1.1 The SEAwall of Institutional Discrimination   14

List of Tables

2.1	Occupational status of visually impaired people, disabled people and non-disabled people	34
2.2	Occupational status following the onset of visual impairment	34
5.1	Degree of sight of the visually impaired physiotherapists	68
5.2	Gender of the sighted and visually impaired physiotherapists	69
5.3	Age of the sighted and visually impaired physiotherapists	70
5.4	Fathers' occupation of the sighted and visually impaired physiotherapists	71
5.5	Mothers' occupation of the sighted and visually impaired physiotherapists	71
5.6	Types of schools attended by the sighted and visually impaired physiotherapists	72
5.7	The views of the sighted and visually impaired physiotherapists on integrated pre-registration education for visually impaired physiotherapy students	73
5.8	Attendance at post-registration courses by the sighted and visually impaired physiotherapists	75
5.9	Types of courses attended by the visually impaired physiotherapists	75
5.10	The degree to which the needs of the visually impaired physiotherapists were met on post-registration courses	76
5.11	The work settings of the sighted and visually impaired physiotherapists	77
5.12	The work specialities of the sighted and visually impaired physiotherapists	78
5.13	Full-time and part-time work of the sighted and visually impaired physiotherapists	79
5.14	Job satisfaction of the sighted and visually impaired physiotherapists	79
5.15	Job satisfaction of the sighted and visually impaired physiotherapists	80
5.16	Choice of physiotherapy as a career for the visually impaired physiotherapists	80
5.17	Satisfaction of the sighted and visually impaired physiotherapists with physiotherapy as a career	81
5.18	Employment grades of the sighted and visually impaired physiotherapists	82

5.19 Promotion prospects of the visually impaired physiotherapists 82
5.20 Number of posts in the careers of the sighted and visually impaired physiotherapists 84
5.21 Perceptions of the attitude of the physiotherapy profession towards visually impaired physiotherapists 85
5.22 The abilities of blind physiotherapists as viewed by the sighted and visually impaired physiotherapists 86
5.23 The abilities of partially sighted physiotherapists as viewed by the sighted and visually impaired physiotherapists 86
5.24 Perceptions of the sighted and visually impaired physiotherapists on the ability of blind physiotherapists to cope in various specialities 87
5.25 Perceptions of the sighted and visually impaired physiotherapists on the ability of partially sighted physiotherapists to cope in various specialities 87
5.26 The perceived suitability of physiotherapy as a career for blind people 89
5.27 The perceived suitability of physiotherapy as a career for partially sighted people 90
5.28 The views of the sighted and visually impaired physiotherapists on the difficulty of physiotherapy as a career for visually impaired people 90

List of Abbreviations

ABCP	Association of Blind Chartered Physiotherapists
AVICP	Association of Visually Impaired Chartered Physiotherapists
BCODP	British Council of Disabled People
CPSM	Council for Professions Supplementary to Medicine
CSP	Chartered Society of Physiotherapy
DPI	Disabled People's International
ISTM	Incorporated Society of Trained Masseuses
ITU	Intensive Care Unit
NHS	National Health Service
NLSP	North London School of Physiotherapy for the Visually Handicapped
PACT	Placement, Assessment and Counselling Teams
RADAR	Royal Association for Disability and Rehabilitation
RNIB	Royal National Institute for the Blind
UPIAS	Union of the Physically Impaired Against Segregation

Introduction

This book and the research upon which it is based, is about disabled people and their employment. It focuses in particular on the barriers disabled people experience at work and the ways in which they overcome, minimise or manage these barriers. It is hoped that this book will provide insights into how disabled people experience and cope with their work at a practical, personal and social level and how changes in legislation, policy and values can impact on their working lives.

Although there are many studies concerning disabled people and employment (see chapter 2), there is very little from the perspective of disabled people themselves (Barnes et al 1998). Kitchin et al state:

> There has been little research to tease out and document the specific mechanisms, structures and processes that underlie disabled people's access to the labour market; or how these processes interact and manifest themselves in different contexts; or an indication of the experiences of disabled people seeking access to the workplace or their experiences within the workplace. (1998: 788)

This book, aims to investigate employment from the direct experiences and perspectives of disabled people themselves. It is based upon a study of visually impaired physiotherapists but it is likely that much of what they experience can be generalised to other disabled people. The book is written from the author's PhD thesis (French 2000) where detail of methodology is given.

Visually Impaired People in the Physiotherapy Profession

Visually impaired people have been accepted for registration by the professional body of physiotherapy (now the Chartered Society of Physiotherapy) since 1916 but have been formally trained since 1895. This can, in many ways, be viewed as an historical accident as physiotherapy developed from massage which visually impaired people traditionally practised (Barclay 1994) (see Chapter 3). Physiotherapy is unique among the professions in recruiting substantial numbers of visually impaired people who, until 1995, received their training in a special college run by the Royal National Institute for the Blind (RNIB). Visually impaired people are, however, employed in other professions including social work and law (Simkiss et al 1998).

The Profession of Physiotherapy

Physiotherapy originated from nursing at the end of the 19th century and originally consisted of treatments using massage. Over the years, however, it has undergone many developments and is now the largest profession supplementary to medicine in Britain with approximately 26,000 people registered as members of the Chartered Society of Physiotherapy (CSP). In the recent career literature of the CSP, physiotherapy is defined as follows:

> *...a healthcare profession which views human movement as central to the health and well-being of individuals. Physiotherapists identify and maximise movement potential through health promotion, preventive health care, treatment and rehabilitation. The core skills used by chartered physiotherapists include manual therapy, therapeutic exercise and the application of electrophysical modalities. Fundamental to the physiotherapist's approach, however, is an appreciation of the psychological, cultural and social factors which influence their clients and the patients' own active role in helping themselves.* (1998: 2)

They go on to say that:

> *Chartered physiotherapists work to combat a range of physical problems, in particular those associated with neuromuscular, musculoskeletal, cardiovascular and respiratory systems.* (1998: 3)

Physiotherapy is a diverse health care profession with opportunities to work in many specialities and many settings. Physiotherapists work within the National Health Service (NHS), special schools, private practice and industry. Specialities include, sports injuries, intensive care, orthopaedics, mental health, learning difficulties, palliative care, paediatrics and neurology. Physiotherapists are also involved in health education and health promotion. This book will focus primarily on visually impaired physiotherapists working within the NHS in a wide variety of specialities.

Physiotherapy became an 'all degree' profession in 1992 and has gradually been transferred from small NHS colleges to the university sector. Courses lead to a B.Sc. Honours degree in Physiotherapy after a three or four year period of study. There is now considerable variation among the courses but they all contain theoretical, practical and clinical components. All the courses are validated, not only by the universities, but by the CSP and the Council for Professions Supplementary to Medicine (CPSM) which administers state registration.

To work within the NHS it is necessary to become State Registered. Once qualified, physiotherapists usually practise as junior physiotherapists for approximately two years within the NHS. They then progress to the grade of Senior 2. In both of these clinical grades physiotherapists usually 'rotate' to different specialities in order to gain wide experience. The top clinical grade within the NHS is that of Senior 1 which many physiotherapists achieve within the first five years of their career. In this grade physiotherapists usually specialise in a particular area and frequently have the responsibility of teaching and assisting junior staff and physiotherapy students.

The higher physiotherapy grades are managerial culminating in the post of District Manager where the post holder manages the physiotherapy services, or the whole rehabilitation service, of an entire health district. The lower managerial grades involve the management of a smaller number of physiotherapists and frequently combine clinical with managerial duties. Many physiotherapists move out of the NHS into private practice or industry and a small minority become lecturers of physiotherapy and move to the university sector.

Physiotherapists are expected to remain active learners throughout their careers and there are a wide variety of courses available from Masters Degrees in Physiotherapy to short courses run by clinical interest groups of the CSP and in-service training. In recent years the CSP has promoted its Professional Development Diary as a tool to document continuing professional development (CSP 1994a). It is likely that continuing professional development will be mandatory within the next few years as it will become necessary for physiotherapists to re-register periodically with the State Registration Board and to do this they will need to show evidence of competence to practise (Physiotherapy 1994a). The Professions Supplementary to Medicine Act (1960) is currently being reviewed with this in mind.

An Outline of the Study

The research on which this book is based was undertaken in two phases over a period of eight years. A survey of visually impaired physiotherapists and sighted physiotherapists was undertaken in 1989–90. Two research tools were used; a questionnaire (involving both the sighted and the visually impaired sample) and semi-structured interviews (involving a proportion of the visually impaired sample only). All the physiotherapists were practising in Britain either privately, in industry, in special schools or within the NHS.

In the questionnaire study the sample of visually impaired physiotherapists was compared with the sample of sighted physiotherapists on a wide range of demographic, personal and employment issues. These data provide a general overview of the employment situation of visually impaired physiotherapists at that time and a comparison of visually impaired physiotherapists with their sighted colleagues.

The 45 semi-structured interviews were based on the individual responses in each research respondent's questionnaire. This data is used in chapter 4 on the history of visually impaired people in the physiotherapy profession, chapter 5 which compares visually impaired physiotherapists with sighted physiotherapists on a wide selection of demographic and work related factors, in chapter 8 on the changing work environment and in chapter 9 where three personal narratives of visually impaired physiotherapists are presented and analysed.

The second phase of the research was undertaken in 1996–97. Twenty of the 45 visually impaired physiotherapists who had been interviewed in phase one of the study were contacted and interviewed again. Only physiotherapists who were working in the NHS were included in this sample although some of them combined this with part-time private work. A semi-structured interview format was used with each respondent with the emphasis on the barriers they experience at work and the strategies they use to overcome, minimise or manage these barriers. People working in private practice were not included as it was decided to focus the study on the experiences of visually impaired physiotherapists working within the NHS which was judged to be an organisation run with the needs of non-disabled employees in mind.

The interviews provide an opportunity to compare the employment situation of the same physiotherapists eight years later which covers a time of considerable change in terms of health and disability legislation, policy and practice. (For full details of the research methodology, readers are referred to French 2000.)

The Rationale for the Study

There are several unique features regarding visually impaired physiotherapists in Britain which makes them an interesting group to study and constitutes an area of research where new insights into disability and employment may be gained. Physiotherapy is the only profession where visually impaired people have, over the course of this century, been accepted in substantial numbers and their special college, which existed from 1915 to 1995, was the only example of a segregated college of higher education in Britain (Teager 1987).

The data from this sample may help to overturn 'taken for granted' assumptions about the ability of disabled people generally, and visually impaired people in particular, to undertake highly skilled, professional work. It is noted in chapter 2 that only approximately 25 per cent of visually impaired people of working age in Britain are employed (Bruce et al 1991) although Simkiss et al (1998), with a smaller sample, give a figure of 32 per cent.

The study is longitudinal, spanning eight years, and many of the physiotherapists had been practising for 20 or 30 years. This provides an historical dimension to the study as the physiotherapists were able to reflect on changes in disability policy and the impact this has had on their employment, changes in health policy and how this has affected their role, changes in themselves as they grow older, and changes in the attitudes and practices within institutions, and within society generally, towards disabled people, for example 'equal opportunity' policies and the impact of the Disability Discrimination Act (DDA) (1995).

The interaction among these and other factors has the potential to provide new insights into the experiences of disabled people at work. 'Equal opportunity' policies and the DDA, for example, have alerted employers and the CSP to the needs and rights of visually impaired physiotherapists, but the NHS and Community Care Act (1990) has created barriers for visually impaired physiotherapists such as an increase in community based practice which requires a high level of mobility and necessitates working in diverse environments. The increased bureaucracy of the NHS has produced more administration which demands new coping strategies from many visually impaired physiotherapists though this may be outweighed by advances in computer technology. This indicates that shifts in policy and values can affect visually impaired physiotherapists, and disabled employees generally, in diverse and unintended ways.

The study is particularly important at the present time as the numbers of disabled people in paid employment is low and they frequently work below their full potential (see chapter 2). It also comes at a time when a Labour government is actively seeking to reduce the number of disabled people who receive state benefits. This is linked to a policy of making people work but which largely ignores the difficulties faced by disabled people seeking paid employment in the open labour market. Fresh insights into the barriers disabled people experience at work and the ways in which they cope with them are urgently required.

A further reason for researching this particular group of people is my own 'insider status'. I have been visually impaired all my life and I trained as a physiotherapist at the RNIB School of Physiotherapy between 1968 and 1972. I therefore have considerable knowledge of visual disability and physiotherapy although I trained as a physiotherapy teacher after just four years of physiotherapy practice.

The Field of Study

The underlying field of study which underpins this book is that of disability studies. Disability studies is a relatively new area of academic enquiry

(Gleeson 1997) which is inter-disciplinary and diverse, drawing on psychology, sociology, linguistics, economics, anthropology, politics, history and media studies (Pfeiffer and Yoshida 1995). Disability studies has been promoted largely by disabled activists and disabled academics from various disciplines, particularly sociology, for example Oliver, Barnes and Shakespeare. There are now several Masters Degree courses in disability studies in Britain and a growing academic literature including the international journal Disability and Society which was launched in 1986. Finkelstein defines disability studies as '...the study of disabled people's lifestyles and aspirations' (1998: 33) and Pfeiffer and Yoshida claim that:

> *The field of disability studies is similar to women's studies and black studies in many ways...Each field focuses upon the individual as well as the societal context.* (1995: 477)

The social model of disability, where disability is defined in terms of barriers external to the person (environmental, structural and attitudinal) lies at the heart of disability studies. The social model of disability is, however, constantly developing and various theorists, for example Morris (1991), Shakespeare et al (1996) and Crow (1996), have attempted to incorporate impairment into the social model of disability and to take account of the individual experiences of disabled people in order to develop a broader model of disability (see chapter 1). This broader conception of the social model of disability will be adopted in this book.

Before the advent of disability studies much of the theoretical analysis of disability took place within medicine and psychology where the voices of disabled people themselves were rarely heard (Oliver 1996a). In this context disability is viewed exclusively in terms of biology and psychological processes and mechanisms; it is regarded as an individual problem rather than a social and political phenomenon (Oliver 1996b, Gleeson 1997).

Outline of the Chapters

This book is divided into three parts; part one explores some theoretical issues which relate to disabled people and employment; part two presents the empirical findings of the research on which the book is based; and part three relates the empirical evidence to the theoretical issues and highlights implications for policy and practice.

Introduction   xvii

Summary of Part 1: Disabled People and Employment: Theoretical Issues

Chapter 1 Models of Disability. This chapter explores two prominent models of disability; the individual model and the social model. The benefits and limitations of these models are explored and the concept of institutional discrimination is examined. This chapter provides a theoretical background for analysing the experiences of the visually impaired physiotherapists.

Chapter 2 Disability and Employment. This chapter gives a broad account of the situation of disabled people in Britain with regard to their employment. It places the experiences of the visually impaired physiotherapists in the context of other visually impaired people and disabled people generally.

Chapter 3 Disabled Health and Welfare Professionals. This chapter presents a literature review of the attitudes of health professionals towards disabled people. It then gives a broad account of the experiences of disabled health and welfare professionals. The chapter provides a context in which to place the visually impaired physiotherapists in relation to other visually impaired health and welfare professionals, for example social workers, and disabled health and welfare professionals generally.

Summary of Part 2: The Experiences of Visually Impaired Physiotherapists

Chapter 4 Visually Impaired Physiotherapists: An Historical Overview. This chapter traces the history of visually impaired people in the physiotherapy profession from the 1890s to the present day. In so doing the history of the CSP is also traced. The chapter provides details of important milestones in the history of visually impaired physiotherapists including the First and Second World Wars and the emergence of the NHS. This chapter includes interview data from phase one of the study.

Chapter 5 A Comparison of Visually Impaired and Sighted Physiotherapists. This chapter uses questionnaire and interview data, collected in phase one of the study, to compare visually impaired and sighted physiotherapists on a number of dimensions including demographic details, work specialities, work settings, promotion prospects, job satisfaction and attitudes to the inclusion of visually impaired physiotherapists in mainstream education. This chapter places the visually impaired physiotherapists within the context of the physiotherapy profession and provides a benchmark with which to compare findings from the second phase of the study.

Chapter 6 Educational Inclusion: Barriers and Coping Strategies. This chapter examines the post-graduate educational experiences of visually impaired physiotherapists. These educational experiences relate to a wide range of courses including higher degrees, short professional courses and in-service training. Data from the semi-structured interviews in the second phase of the study are used in this analysis.

Chapter 7 Employment: Barriers and Coping Strategies. This chapter explores the barriers visually impaired physiotherapists experience at work and the strategies they use to overcome or minimise these barriers. It draws on a thematic analysis of the interview data undertaken in the second phase of the study.

Chapter 8 The Changing Work Environment: Its Impact on Visually Impaired Physiotherapists. This chapter considers how changes in legislation, policy and practice, in both health care and disability, have impacted upon the working lives of visually impaired physiotherapists. It also gives the physiotherapists an opportunity to reflect on their careers in terms, for example, of their job satisfaction and promotion. The chapter draws upon interview data from both phases of the study.

Chapter 9 Personal Narratives: Disabling Barriers – Enabling Contexts. This chapter presents narratives of three of the visually impaired physiotherapists drawing on both phases of the study. The aim of this chapter is to present three visually impaired physiotherapists who have pursued different careers within physiotherapy and who have perceived and approached barriers in different ways. The presentation of 'whole stories' serves to balance the thematic analysis which considers themes across all of the interviews. The narratives highlight the complexity of barriers and coping strategies in the lives of different people in diverse circumstances.

Summary of Part 3: Overview and Concluding Comments

Chapter 10 Discussion and Conclusion. This chapter assesses and interprets the major findings of the study in the light of the literature review presented in Part One of the book. The contribution that the book makes to the field of disability studies is examined and the implications of the book for policy and practice with regard to the employment of visually impaired people, and disabled people generally, is discussed.

PART 1

DISABLED PEOPLE AND EMPLOYMENT: THEORETICAL ISSUES

Chapter 1

Models of Disability

In the first part of this chapter two central models of disability will be discussed; the individual model and the social model. There are other models of disability, for example those derived from religion where disability may be regarded as a gift or a punishment (Barnes 1992, Hughes 1998, Stiker 1999) but these no longer have a strong influence in British society. They do indicate, however, that disability (and indeed impairment) are socially constructed and can change in meaning over time and across cultures.

Towards the end of this chapter the concept of institutional discrimination will be examined. The concept of institutional discrimination in relation to disabled people (institutional disablism) has been articulated by disabled people themselves and has been influenced by the social model of disability. As Priestley states:

> *The disabled people's movement has struggled hard to gain acceptance for the idea that disability can be considered as a form of institutional discrimination or collective social oppression.* (1999: 9)

Institutional discrimination analyses oppression within institutions in terms of attitudinal, environmental, cultural and structural barriers (Thompson 1997, Swain et al 1998). The social model of disability also focuses on external barriers rather than looking for limitations and solutions within disabled people themselves.

What is a Model?

The terms 'theory' and 'model' are often used interchangeably. Polgar and Thomas define theories as:

> *...conjectures representing our current state of knowledge about the world...a theory will clarify the relationships between diverse classes of observations and hypotheses.* (1995: 6–7)

They define models, in contrast, as representing specific aspects of a theory.

Within every society there are competing models of disability with some being more dominant than others at different times (Finkelstein 1993,

French 1997a, Hughes 1998). These models although often in conflict, gradually influence and modify each other. The models put forward by powerful groups within society, such as the medical profession, tend to dominate the models of less powerful groups, such as those of disabled people themselves (Finkelstein 1993, Oliver 1996b).

It is essential to explore these models of disability for attitudes and behaviour towards disabled people, policy, professional practice, and the running of institutions, including places of employment, are based, at least in part, upon them. As Oliver states:

> The 'lack of fit' between able-bodied and disabled people's definitions is more than just a semantic quibble for it has important implications both for the provision of services and the ability to control one's life. (1993a: 61)

The Individual Model of Disability

The most widespread view of disability at the present time is based upon the assumption that the difficulties disabled people experience are a direct result of their individual physical, sensory or intellectual impairments (Oliver and Sapey 1999, Priestley 1999). Thus the blind person who falls down a hole in the pavement does so because he or she failed to see it, and the person with a motor impairment fails to get into the building because of his or her inability to walk. Problems are thus viewed as residing within the individual (Swain et al 1993, Hales 1996). The individual model of disability is deeply ingrained and 'taken as given' in the medical, psychological and sociological literature though various composite models have been developed, for example the biopsychosocial model (Cooper et al 1996). Priestley refers to the tendency to individualise disability as the 'culture of embodiment' which he also relates to other oppressed groups:

> The legitimacy of individual models of disability is premised upon the assumption that the disadvantage experienced by disabled people is a product of the 'imperfect' body...in this respect there is a striking similarity with the way in which cultural representation of women and black people have contributed to the maintenance of their oppression...The pejorative scaling of bodies under the normalising gaze of biological science, has persistently identified black people and women with undesirable bodily attributes. (1999: 34–5)

The medical model can be regarded as a sub-category of the over-arching individual model of disability where disability is conceived as part of the disease process, abnormality and individual tragedy – something which happens to unfortunate individuals on a more or less random basis. The problems disabled people encounter are seen to lie within the disabled person rather than within society. Disabled people are, for example, frequently critical of the countless hours spent attempting to learn to walk at the expense of their education or leisure (Sutherland 1981, Oliver 1996b). The individual model of disability may, therefore, be viewed as taking a 'victim blaming' stance (Ryan 1976) which has also been applied to other oppressed groups including those of low socio-economic status (Ryan 1976) and people in developing countries (Allen and Thomas 2000).

None of these arguments imply that considering the medical or individual needs of disabled individuals is wrong; the argument is that the individual model of disability has tended to view disability only in those terms focusing almost exclusively on attempting to modify people's impairments and returning them or approximating them to 'normal'. The effect of the physical, attitudinal and social environment on disabled people has tended to be regarded as relatively fixed which has maintained the status quo keeping disabled people in their disadvantaged state within society (Oliver and Sapey 1999). Thus the onus is on disabled people to adapt to a disabling environment (Swain et al 1993, Hales 1996, French et al 1997). This is something which disabled people and their allies are increasingly challenging. Oliver states:

> *The disability movement throughout the world is rejecting approaches based upon the restoration of normality and insisting on approaches based upon the celebration of difference.* (1996b: 44)

Morris (1991) believes that there is a need to celebrate difference whilst maintaining solidarity against the commonality of oppression.

Individualistic definitions of disability certainly have the potential to do serious harm. The medicalisation of learning disabilities, whereby people were institutionalised and abused, is one example (Ryan and Thomas 1987, 1990, Potts and Fido 1991, Atkinson et al 2000). Another is 'sight saving' classes in schools where visually impaired children were prevented from using their sight (Corley et al 1989). Disabled children have been categorised into schools according to their impairments, where they have been segregated from society, frequently abused, and usually given an inferior education (Barnes 1991, Humphries and Gordon 1992, French 1996, French and Swain 2000).

Oliver (1993b) is of the opinion that the individual model of disability may serve the needs of professionals more than the needs of disabled people. Wendell is also suspicious of the involvement of professionals in the lives of disabled people. She states:

> *...both the charities and most government bureaucracies...hand out help which would not be needed in a society that was planned and organised to include*

people with a wide range of physical and mental abilities. The potential resistance created by these vested interests in disability should not be under-estimated. (1996: 53)

By individualising disability the effect of the environment upon the lives of disabled people is not addressed. Indeed the environments imposed upon disabled people in the name of treatment, for example mental handicap hospitals and special schools, can have detrimental effects leading to greater dependency and an increase in existing problems of function or behaviour (Potts and Fido 1991, French 1996). Finkelstein and Stuart (1996) are of the opinion that issues relating to disability would be better placed in the Department of the Environment, rather than the Department of Health, and that important new disciplines in engineering and architecture need to be developed in order to make the environment more accessible to disabled people.

Within the individual model, disability is viewed as an individual tragedy to which disabled people must 'adjust' (Thompson 1997, Oliver and Sapey 1999). The period of adjustment is frequently depicted in terms of the typical stages of grief (denial, anger, depression and acceptance) which were outlined by Kubler-Ross (1969) in relation to terminal illness. According to Oliver and Sapey (1999) non-disabled people have imagined what it must be like to be disabled, have assumed it would be a tragedy and have decided that it would require a difficult psychological adjustment. The social model, on the other hand, views adjustment as a task for society rather than the individual disabled person and, while recognising that disability may be a cause of psychological distress, refutes the suggestion that this is inevitably the case.

As well as the external oppression disabled people experience from disabling environments and other people's attitudes and expectations, disabled people can also become internally oppressed by viewing themselves in the same way as many non-disabled people view them, and behaving as others expect them to behave (Goffman 1968, Oliver and Barnes 1998). Woolley explains:

We are oppressed from without by a society which does not value us and therefore does not give priority to our needs, and we are oppressed from within because we have internalised these same attitudes towards ourselves. (1993: 81)

This self-fulfilling prophecy can, in turn, lead to 'proof' that the erroneous attitudes and beliefs about disabled people are correct which can serve to justify the treatment they receive creating a vicious circle (Finkelstein and French 1993). Wolfensberger and Tullman contend that 'The social roles that people impose on each other or adopt are among the most powerful social influences and control methods known' (1989: 215).

It is not at all surprising that disabled people internalise the views of the wider society as, with the exception of the indigenous deaf community (those who are born deaf) there has been very little sense of cultural identity among them until recent times. This makes it difficult for disabled people to reject the expectations and beliefs, about how they should think, feel and behave, which other people may hold. Disabled children, in particular, are very vulnerable to this conditioning. Their parents are often unwitting oppressors in the process, with their beliefs and expectations being shaped by those of professional 'experts' and society at large (Oliver and Barnes 1998). As Morris states:

> *Most of the people we have dealings with, including our most intimate relationships, are not like us. It is therefore very difficult for us to recognise and challenge the values and judgements that are applied to us and our lives. Our ideas about disability and about ourselves are generally formed by those who are not disabled.* (1991: 37)

These disabling expectations and attitudes are, however, rarely completely internalised. It can also be entirely rational to behave in ways which other people expect in order, for example, to gain support or approval (French 1993a). Such ways of behaving can, nevertheless, give rise to passivity, anxiety and depression (Goffman 1968) and many disabled people spend a great deal of time and energy attempting to reverse their social conditioning (Sutherland 1981, Woolley 1993).

The Social Model of Disability

The social model of disability is often referred to as the 'barriers approach' where disability is viewed, not in terms of the individual's impairment, but in terms of environmental, structural, and attitudinal barriers which impinge upon the lives of disabled people, and which have the potential to impede their inclusion and progress in many areas of life, including employment, unless they are minimised or removed (Lonsdale 1985, Oliver 1996b, French and Swain 1997, French et al 1997). The social model of disability has arisen from the thinking and writings of disabled people themselves (Oliver and Sapey 1999). As Priestley asserts, '...the development of the disabled people's movement is inextricably bound up with a social model of disability' (1999: 35).

An Outline of the Disabled People's Movement

Before exploring the social model of disability in more detail, it is necessary to place it within its historical context within the disabled people's movement and to examine briefly the origins and growth of that movement. The disabled people's movement comprises the collective thoughts, actions and experiences of disabled people themselves.

Social movements arise as a result of specific or widespread grievances and unrest; their goal is usually to reorganise society in some fundamental way (Abercrombie 1988). Social movements have been defined by Giddens as:

> ...a collective attempt to further a common interest, or secure a common goal, through collective action outside the sphere of established institutions. (1989: 624)

They are led and controlled primarily by oppressed people themselves when, through sharing their experiences with similar people, they come to attribute the source of their concerns to social conditions and seek to find political solutions. Davis, talking of the disabled people's movement, states:

> The movement came when disabled individuals first faced up to the fact that they could achieve more for themselves through collective action than they could on their own. (1993a: 287)

Oliver (1996b) places the disabled people's movement among the 'new social movements' which have emerged during the second half of the twentieth century; the women's movement, the black civil rights movement, Gay Pride and Mad Pride are other examples. The aim of these movements is to gain equality and social justice.

The disabled people's movement comprises organisations *of* disabled people. Organisations *of* disabled people are those where disabled people are in positions of control. Although such groups have proliferated in recent years, it is a mistake to imagine that the resistance of disabled people to oppression is a recent phenomenon. Two early organisations of this type in Britain were the British Deaf Association (founded in 1890) and The National League of the Blind (founded in 1899). These early groups were militant, focusing on the particular problems deaf and blind people faced within an environment designed for non-disabled living. Other social movements, for example the women's movement, were also active at this time (Summerfield 1996).

Over the next 60 years, many other organisations of disabled people developed. They usually focused on specific impairments or single issues, such as lack of state provision. The National Federation of the Blind, for example, was formed in 1947. During the 1960s and 1970s, organisations of disabled people which crossed impairment boundaries began to develop; the issue which drew them together was poverty. The Disablement Income Group (DIG), formed in 1965, for example, aimed to secure a disability allowance from the state for all disabled people to compensate them for the extra costs of disability; its appeals and campaigns were notably unsuccessful.

Perhaps the most significant turning point for the disabled people's movement in Britain was the formation in 1974 of the Union of the Physically Impaired Against Segregation (UPIAS). Davis (1993a) explains how UPIAS fought to change the definition of disability from one of individual tragedy to one of social oppression. This paved the way for the development of the social model of disability which is at the intellectual heart of the disabled people's movement (Priestley 1999) and is referred to by Hasler (1993) as the 'big idea'. The Liberation Network of Disabled People, which was led by disabled women, also developed at this time. It challenged disabling barriers at a more personal level focusing, for example, on internal oppression and denial of disability (Campbell and Oliver 1996). It provided a less overtly political forum for the discussion of ideas and experiences.

In 1981 a group of disabled activists came together to form the British Council of Organisations of Disabled People (BCODP) which is an umbrella group for organisations of disabled people. A large number of BCODP's member organisations comprise coalitions of disabled people and Centres of Integrated Living which offer a range of services for disabled people and are run and controlled by disabled people themselves. Other member organisations include those which focus on specific impairments or single issues, for example GEMMA (an organisation of disabled lesbians) and The Association of Blind Asians.

During the 1980s BCODP grew and continues to expand; in 1999 it represented 123 organisations and 350,000 disabled people, and is recognised as the representative voice of disabled people in Britain. It articulates its demands through formal political channels and lobbies and advises both central and local government. It undertakes research and organises and supports demonstrations and campaigns of direct action. In 1997 it changed its name to the British Council of Disabled People (BCODP) as individual disabled people can now join.

Disabled People's International (DPI) was also formed in 1981. It is an international umbrella group of organisations of disabled people. In 1999 it represented 113 national assemblies of disabled people, including BCODP, and is recognised by the United Nations as the representative voice of disabled people internationally.

An important element in the struggle of disabled people for equality and social justice, is the disability arts movement. Disability arts have the power to communicate the distinctive history, skills, customs, life-styles, experiences, and concerns of disabled people. Disability arts are mainly directed at disabled people themselves. Most gatherings of disabled people, such as demonstrations, include disabled artists – singers, writers, painters, comedians – who express the experience of disability from their own perspectives, providing alternative, positive, and often overtly political ways of viewing disability and society.

The Origin of The Social Model of Disability

The social model of disability has arisen directly from the disabled people's movement and the growing cultural identity of disabled people. This radical interpretation of disability offers disabled people affirmation and support as they re-define their situation. In the past it has been thought unnecessary to discover how disabled people view the circumstances of their lives. Very little had been written by disabled people themselves until the 1980s but with the growth of the disabled people's movement and the introduction of disability studies as an academic discipline in universities, this situation has changed. Oliver states:

> *From the 1950s onwards there was a growing realisation that if particular social problems were to be resolved, or at least ameliorated, then nothing more or less than a fundamental redefinition of the problem was necessary.* (1990: 3)

The following definition of impairment and disability is that of the Union of the Physically Impaired Against segregation. The major importance of this definition is that it breaks the link between impairment and disability:

> *Impairment*
> *Lacking part or all of a limb, or having a defective limb, organ or mechanism of the body.*
>
> *Disability*
> *The disadvantage or restriction of activity caused by a contemporary social organisation which takes no or little account of people who have physical impairments and thus excludes them from participation in the mainstream of social activities. Physical disability is therefore a particular form of social oppression.* (UPIAS 1976: 14)

The word 'physical' is now frequently removed from this definition so as to include people with learning difficulties and survivors of the mental health system (Oliver and Barnes 1998). This, and similar later definitions, break the connection between impairment and disability which are viewed as separate entities with no causal link. This is similar to the distinction made between sex (a biological entity) and gender (a social entity) in the women's movement (Saraga 1998).

Disability is viewed within the social model of disability in terms of barriers (Swain et al 1993). There are three types of barriers which all interact:

1. Structural barriers – which refer to the underlying norms, mores and ideologies of organisations and institutions which are based on judgements of 'normality' and which are sustained by hierarchies of power.
2. Environmental barriers – which refer to physical barriers within the environment, for example steps, holes in the pavement, and lack of resources for disabled people, for example lack of braille and lack of sign language interpreters. It also refers to the ways things are done which may exclude disabled people, for example the way meetings are conducted and the time allowed for tasks.
3. Attitudinal barriers – which refer to the adverse attitudes and behaviour of people towards disabled people.

The social model of disability locates disability, not within the individual disabled person, but within society. Thus the person who uses a wheelchair is not disabled by paralysis but by building design, lack of lifts, rigid work practices, and the attitudes and behaviour of others. Similarly the visually impaired person is not disabled by lack of sight, but by lack of braille, cluttered pavements, and stereotypical ideas about blindness. Finkelstein (1981, 1998) has argued that non-disabled people would be equally disabled if the environment was not designed with their needs in mind. Human beings fashion the world to suit their own capabilities and limitations and disabled people are wanting nothing more than that.

Attitudinal barriers are regarded within the social model of disability as very significant but only in the context of environmental and structural barriers (Swain et al 1998). It is believed that an exclusive focus on attitudes will never be successful yet this is where most focus lies (Swain and Lawrence 1994). This can be seen in the government's various campaigns to change the attitudes of employers, which have been notoriously unsuccessful, and its great reluctance over the years to introduce comprehensive disability discrimination legislation. Oliver contends that 'Discrimination does not exist in the prejudiced attitudes of individuals but in the institutionalised practices of society' (1996b: 76). If the focus is solely on the attitudes and behaviour of individuals then the structural and environmental barriers, and the power structures which maintain them, are ignored.

The social model of disability arises from the collective experiences of disabled people themselves. It has engendered personal and political empowerment, self-confidence and pride (Morris 1991). Hevey, for example, describes his introduction to the social model of disability as 'a flash on the road to Damascus' (1992: 1) and Crow states:

> *For years now the social model of disability has enabled me to confront, survive and even surmount countless situations of exclusion and discrimination. It has been my mainstay as it has been for the wider Disabled People's Movement. It has enabled a view of ourselves free from the constraints of disability (oppression) and has provided a direction for our commitment to social change. It has played a central role in promoting disabled people's individual self-worth, collective identity and political organisation.* (1996: 207)

Disabled people are thus engaged in a struggle to replace the individual model of disability with a model couched in terms of civil rights. Oliver talks of its considerable success:

> *For the past 15 years the social model of disability has been the foundation upon which disabled people have chosen to organise themselves collectively. This has resulted in unparalleled success in changing the discourse around disability, in promoting disability as a civil rights issue and in developing schemes to give disabled people autonomy and control in their own lives.* (1996b: 40)

One of its achievements was the passing, in 1995, of the Disability Discrimination Act after many years of campaigning. This act is, however, far from comprehensive and cannot be regarded as full civil rights legislation (see chapter 2).

Institutional Discrimination

Swain et al define institutional discrimination as:

> *Unfair or unequal treatment of individuals or groups which is built into institutional organisations, policies and practices at personal, environmental and structural levels.* (Swain et al 1998: 5)

Disabled people face institutional discrimination in a social and physical world that is geared by, for and towards non-disabled people. The notion of institutional discrimination has played an important role in the development of disability theory (Barnes 1991) generating from a social model of disability and developed by disabled people themselves. The commonalties in issues of racism, sexism, homophobia and disablism can be explored through themes such as attitudes, power relationships, the denial of rights and discriminatory language, while also highlighting differences in the

forms of discrimination faced by different groups (T...
   Essential to understanding discrimination as b...
reject individualised, or victim blaming explan...
To see discrimination as institutional is to re...
woven into the very structure and fabric of b...
organisations such as places of employment.
   People with impairments are disabled by institu...
prevent their full participative citizenship within society an...
and participation within organisations. Figure 1.1 the ...
Institutional Discrimination, depicts these barriers as the bricks in a...
this model of institutional discrimination, attitudinal barriers are constru...
on environmental barriers which are themselves founded on structural barri...
ers. Ideology plays a key role in the inter-reliance between each layer (Swain et al 1998).

At the structural level, institutional discrimination is built into what might be called the macro-systems of British society: economic, education and welfare. Oliver (1991) and Finkelstein (1993) both argue that disabled people are largely excluded from labour market participation because of changes in the work processes that came with the coming of our industrialised, capitalist society which insists on speed and competition. Many disabled people have also been excluded from mainstream educational provision which has had the effect of reducing their subsequent life chances in terms of employment and wealth (Barnes 1991). In recent years the concept of citizenship has been drawn upon in understanding structural barriers (Oliver 1996b). Disabled people, as a group, are denied political, social and human rights that many non-disabled people take for granted.

The hierarchy of social divisions is built into institutions and organisations through formal arrangements that govern social interaction among people. These formal arrangements, such as fire regulations, rigid timetables and assessment and examination procedures, create environmental barriers which can restrict certain groups of people including disabled people. Discrimination is also encountered by disabled people in their daily interactions with the physical world of transport, housing and equipment, and physical barriers, such as cars parked on the pavement and the position of furniture in a classroom. Equipment is geared to the needs and norms of non-disabled people (for example steps, taps, cars, buses) with the needs of disabled people being marginalised as 'special'. The picture is complex in that the needs of disabled people are diverse (for instance a lack of curbs is advantageous to people who use wheelchairs but is problematic for blind people who use them to distinguish between the pavement and the road). However, non-disabled norms take little account of such human diversity.

Cemented by ideologies of 'normality' and 'independence'

ATTITUDINAL	**Cognitive prejudice:** assumptions about the (in)abilities, emotional responses and needs of disabled people	**Emotional prejudice:** fear	**Behavioural prejudice:** individual practice and praxis
ENVIRONMENTAL	**Disablist language**	**Institutional policies, organisation, rules and regulations**	**Professional practices:** assessment, care management	**Inaccessible physical environments**
STRUCTURAL	**Hierarchical power relations and structures:** the disempowerment of disabled people	**The denial of human, social and welfare rights**	**Structural inequalities:** poverty

Reproduced with acknowledgement from Swain et al. 1998

Source: Swain, J., Gillman, M. and French, S. (1998), Confronting Disabling Barriers: Towards Making Organisations Accessible, Venture Press, Birmingham, p. 5.

Figure 1.1   The SEAwall of Institutional Discrimination

Attitudinal discrimination refers to negative feelings, beliefs and behaviours towards disabled people. Attitudes are complex. They are generally seen as having three components: a cognitive component, that is knowledge and understanding of disability; an emotional component, that is the feelings provoked by disabled people; a behavioural component, that is how people act and react towards disabled people (Fishbein and Ajken 1975). Attitudes are complicated further because there is a loose connection among these three components. People's understandings, feelings and behaviour do not necessarily relate closely to each other. Nevertheless, each of the three components is seen to play a part in negative attitudes. A negative attitude towards visually impaired people might include a lack of understanding about visual impairment, fear of visually impaired people and negative labelling which may, in turn, lead to discrimination in, for example, employment. The concept of institutional discrimination is related to the social model of disability in that both emphasise the ways in which external barriers create disability.

Conclusion

This chapter has explored the individual and the social models of disability. The concept of institutional discrimination was also introduced as it provides a framework for understanding many of the problems disabled people experience within organisations, including their places of work. The following chapter will give a broad overview of the employment situation of disabled people in general, and visually impaired people in particular, in Britain today. This will provide a context for examining the particular situation of the visually impaired physiotherapists presented in Part Two of this book and will be drawn upon to analyse their experiences.

Chapter 2

Disability and Employment

There is nothing at all in disability as such that says that people who live with it can't work. (Shearer 1981: 156)

This chapter aims to document the overall employment situation of disabled people in Britain today. It will also give a specific account of the employment position of visually impaired people. This will help to set in context the employment of visually impaired physiotherapists, which forms the basis of the study presented in Part 2 of this book, and to provide a framework against which their experiences will be analysed.

Employment and Unemployment

Disabled people are far more likely to be unemployed than non-disabled people, and are highly represented among the long term unemployed (Barnes et al 1998). Sixty per cent of disabled people in most industrialised countries are out of work (Hahn 1997). In 1999 disabled people made up half of those who were unemployed but said they would like to work (Burchardt 2000).

This situation exists despite the 1944 Employment Act where most companies employing 20 or more people were obliged to ensure that three per cent of the workforce comprised registered disabled people if they were available for work. This law was not, however, enforced. In 1992 just 20 per cent of employers met the quota, and only ten prosecutions have ever been made, with none being made since 1975 (RADAR 1993). Prescott-Clarke (1990) found that many disabled people had never heard of the scheme and that 26 per cent believed that registration made it more difficult to get a job. The scheme was abandoned in 1996 with the introduction of the Disability Discrimination Act in 1995.

It is clear, however, that many disabled people are quite capable of working if given the opportunity to do so. In 1986 Lambeth Council decided to reserve all new posts within the council for disabled people; they rapidly recruited 200 disabled people and greatly exceeded the three per cent employment quota (Disability – Changing Practice 1990).

The employment of disabled people, like that of women, fluctuates with wider social and economic circumstances. If there is a shortage in the labour force disabled people are more likely to find work (Burchardt 2000). This situation arose during the first few months of the second world war when 400,000 disabled people, who were previously unemployed, were given work only to lose it when the war ended (Humphreys and Gordon 1992, Hahn 1997). As Clarke and Saraga point out:

> *Employability (or the lack of it) is a social characteristic rather than a personal attribute. It sums up a variety of social judgements about what sorts of people make desirable employees, and these judgements change over time and between societies.* (1998: 1)

Three per cent of the work force become disabled each year and many disabled people lose their jobs at the onset of impairment (Barnes et al 1998). Morris (1989) reports that of 103 women who were in full-time employment before their spinal cord injuries, 48 did not return to work, 39 took up a different type of employment, and 15 changed to part-time work. Some felt they could not or did not want to compete and deliberately opted out of the employment market.

The incidence of impairment increases with age and disabled people, like other people, are subject to ageism as well as disablism when seeking employment (French 1997b, Barnes et al 1998, Thompson 1998). Simkiss et al (1998) found that the highest rate of employment for visually impaired people was between the ages of 26 and 40. This confirms evidence cited by Simkiss et al (1998) which shows that disability exaggerates a tendency to push older people into unemployment. Employment rates among disabled people who are over 50 are particularly low (Burchardt 2000).

Burchardt (2000) points out that if disabled people find employment it tends to be poorly paid, and Roulstone states that:

> *Not only are disabled people much more likely to be denied the chance to work, but even when employment is achieved, they are less likely to attain high status employment relative to the general population.* (1998: 34)

The positive correlation between disability and both low pay and low occupational status is very marked, with disabled people being over-represented in unskilled and semi-skilled occupations (Barnes et al 1998). Simkiss et al state, in relation to their survey of visually impaired people, that:

> *There is overwhelming evidence that blind and partially sighted people secure fewer opportunities in their employment than their educational achievements should lead them to expect.* (1998: 12)

Disabled people are more likely to be in part-time or temporary work and to work within small, rather than large, organisations. They are also more likely than non-disabled people to work from home.

Despite the reluctance to employ disabled people, there is some evidence to suggest that they are more efficient and competent than other employees, that they stay longer in a job, take less sick leave, and are more conscientious (Local Government Management Board 1991). Kettle (1979) reviewed many studies of disabled employees which indicated these trends. Greenwood and Johnson (1987) reviewed the literature on the employment of disabled people from the 1940s to the 1980s in the USA. They found that absenteeism and turnover were equal or lower than that of non-disabled workers and that the productivity of disabled workers was equally as good. Similar findings are reported by The Royal Association for Disability and Rehabilitation (RADAR) (1993) who found that disabled workers were equal or better than non-disabled workers on productivity, attitude to work, and attendance. Balser and Harvey (1993) found that disabled people working in hospitals had no higher accident rates or turnover than average, took no more sick leave than other workers, and were no more difficult to train; in many instances their work record was superior to that of their non-disabled colleagues.

The good work record of disabled people may reflect a lack of employment opportunities, as well as real or perceived feelings of vulnerability. This may lead disabled people to try to 'compensate' for disability (Goffman 1968, Barnes 1996). The emphasis on being 'as good' or 'better than' non-disabled workers is oppressive to many disabled people. Barnes et al found in their interviews with disabled people that:

> *Some people commented on the pressures on them to sustain the image of the more loyal, hard-working and conscientious employee which is widely promoted in government propaganda and subscribed to by some organisations of and for disabled people.* (1998: 20)

Oliver and Barnes conclude that:

> *Expecting severely disabled people to be as productive as non-disabled people is one of the most oppressive aspects of capitalist society.* (1998: 96)

The Social and Psychological Benefits of Work

> *The opportunity to gain employment is one of the most significant factors affecting the life of a disabled person. Employment opens up the prospect of financial independence and the possibility of a rewarding career. The challenges and rewards of work are taken for granted by a large part of the population. Yet the*

> *experience of many disabled people has shown that the process of trying to gain employment is one of consistent discrimination against them on the grounds of their disability.* (Graham et al 1990: 1)

Paid employment has the potential to bring many social and psychological benefits to people who engage in it (Barnes et al 1998). This is not to imply that paid employment is the only route to satisfaction; it is quite possible to gain equal social and psychological benefits from work or leisure which is unpaid (Barnes et al 1998, Burchardt 2000). However, in British society at the present time, being in paid employment is given great value and status, and many people, including disabled people, who cannot find work suffer socially and psychologically as a result. Prescott-Clarke (1990) found more mental health problems among unemployed disabled people than those who worked. Lack of work also leads to lack of resources, so that people cannot afford to do many of the things that bring them pleasure. Oliver and Barnes state that:

> *...in our view, it is the exclusion from the world of work which is the ultimate cause of the various other exclusions experienced by disabled people.* (1998: 95)

Lonsdale (1990) argues that work structures the day and provides company, friendship, and dignity, and Shearer states that it is 'a passport to the adult world' (1981: 158). Being in paid employment may give status and security, increased self-confidence, and a feeling of being useful to society. According to the individual's temperament and circumstances, unemployment can give rise to boredom, isolation and lack of confidence. Many disabled people regard paid employment as a major aspect of their struggle for equality (Abberley 1996). As well as the many personal and social benefits employment can bring it also provides an income which can help to counter some of the many barriers disabled people face (Zarb 1995a).

Sutherland points out that lack of employment can mean lack of power. Talking of disabled people he states:

> *As an economic force we are at present insignificant, there is little opportunity of our 'holding the country to ransom' – would that we could!...Equality of opportunity would enable us to start to acquire some degree of economic leverage, which would mean that our voices would be likely to be listened to rather more than they are at present.* (1981: 33)

Although work can be seen to be very important, both in a psychological and social sense, Lonsdale (1990) points out that by holding down a job disabled people may sacrifice other aspects of their lives; they may, for example, need to use all their leisure time and energy to keep pace with their work. This is exacerbated by the vulnerability disabled people feel which leads to a need to 'compensate' for being disabled (Barnes 1996). Shearer quotes a blind woman as saying:

> *I feel I have to be really good, not ill often and always producing my best. I don't want to give anyone the chance to criticise me or to think I cannot cope because of being blind, it can be quite exhausting.* (1981: 45)

The issue of time is important for visually impaired employees as their reading and working speeds are slower than those of their non-disabled colleagues. It is considerably slower to read braille than it is for sighted people to read print although variable speed tape recorders do allow for greater reading speeds than can be achieved with braille (McCall 1994) In addition, as Dodds points out, reading 'involves the person in a lot of effort. Great amounts of concentration are required to extract useful information and this is tiring' (1993: 34). Baron et al (1996) point out that most disabled people, regardless of impairment, needs more time to carry out tasks.

Thompson (1998) points out that discrimination and oppression at work can be significant sources of stress and that those who are low in the occupational hierarchy have less access to support or resources to help them cope. The relationship between work and well-being is thus far from clear (Barnes et al 1998).

Barriers to Employment

Environmental and Structural Barriers

Some of the unemployment of disabled people results from difficulties not directly related to the job itself and can be explained in terms of barriers and institutional disablism (Barnes et al 1998). In his study of disabled men in Lambeth, West (1989) found that 21 per cent experienced barriers to travel, and Lonsdale (1990) points out that disabled people tend to have to travel further to find work, perhaps to a local authority with progressive equal opportunity policies. Morris (1989) found that the disabled women she interviewed complained of physical access barriers, and Barnes (1991) and Zarb (1995a) speak of unadapted public transport and buildings, and restrictive safety regulations.

The environment can, of course, be adapted and people are beginning to accept the idea that disabled people should not be solely responsible for managing disability, but rather that it should be regarded as a social and political phenomenon (Swain et al 1993, Campbell and Oliver 1996). Talking of visual impairment Bradfield states:

> *While much emphasis has been placed on the acquisition of basic skills required to perform tasks, it has become increasingly obvious that the impact of external or environmental factors plays an important role in the ability of the worker to perform the job. In fact, these factors, if not attended to, may prohibit otherwise qualified workers from obtaining employment.* (1992: 39)

At the present time, however, the social organisation of work leads to considerable insensitivity to, and lack of awareness of, the barriers which disabled people face and how this may exclude them from paid employment or minimise their chances of promotion (Smith 1996). The working environment may also have become more difficult for disabled people. Recent changes include a decrease in unskilled work, the rapid development of technology and the necessity to be multi-skilled and to adapt to rapidly changing environments (Barnes et al 1998). Wendell states:

> *When the pace of life in a society increases, there is a tendency for more people to become disabled, not only because of physically damaging consequences of efforts to go faster, but also because fewer people can meet expectations of 'normal' performance.* (1996: 37)

Intellectual skills have also became more important thus disadvantaging people with learning difficulties and those who have not had the advantage of an extensive education, which includes many disabled people.

Although disabled people encounter specific barriers to employment they share many of these barriers with non-disabled people for example lack of personal transport, poor education and low socio-economic status. Burchardt states:

> *Employment opportunities for disabled people are influenced by many of the same trends as for the rest of the population but, often, disabled people are more severely affected.* (2000: 27)

Attitudinal Barriers

Many disabled people find that employers are prejudiced and discriminate against them (Roulstone 1998, Barnes et al 1998, Simkiss et al 1998). Barnes et al, talking of their interviews with disabled people, state:

> *The need to confront stereotypical views held by employers emerged as an important strand in discussion. Perceptions about costs, for instance, are often based on misguided notions of the types of workplace adjustments which are required.* (1998: 42)

Some of the disabled women Morris (1989) interviewed mentioned blatant and overt discrimination and prejudice; for example, a doctor who sustained a spinal cord injury found that her two partners would not accept her back in the practice, although she found a satisfactory position elsewhere. Wendell states:

> Most able-bodied people cannot wrap their minds around the possibility that someone can be disabled and ill and also work productively...Thus they infer that someone who can work at all cannot be significantly disabled. (1996: 4)

Dyer (1990) found that a third of the 26 health authorities sampled chose not to employ disabled people, and Chinnery (1990) found that non-disabled workers regularly engage in discriminatory behaviour including open hostility. Barnes (1991) and Barnes et al (1998) point out that disabled people may be discriminated against in terms of their appearance, as they may not promote a particular image. This may be particularly so when people are working directly with the public. It was a factor in the attitudes of physiotherapists to the recruitment of hypothetical disabled colleagues (French 1987).

It is pointed out by RADAR (1993) that many employers believe that their field of employment is unsuitable for disabled people. This belief is probably reinforced by the absence of disabled people in the workforce. Many employers feel that they cannot afford disabled workers and yet most disabled people do not need extensive modifications, and if they do government help may be available (Barnes 1991, Roulstone 1998).

In a study by Fry (1986) for the Spastics Society (now Scope), pairs of letters were sent applying for secretarial posts in London. The letters were the same except in one the person said that she had cerebral palsy but that it did not interfere with her ability to work. Almost all of the jobs were in the private sector. Ninety seven per cent of the non-disabled applicants received positive replies compared with only 59 per cent of the disabled applicants. This places disabled people in a dilemma about whether or not to reveal their impairments (French 1997c, Barnes et al 1998). Simkiss et al (1998) found that four out of five visually impaired people disclosed their impairments when applying for jobs although many were in a dilemma about whether or not it was wise to do so.

A similar study was undertaken for the Spastics Society by Graham et al (1990) with comparable results. Of the 94 employers who responded positively to both or either of the fictitious applicants, 88 offered interviews to the non-disabled applicants and 57 to the disabled applicants; thus six of the non-disabled applicants were rejected compared with 37 of the disabled applicants. The employers were found to impose restrictions on the disabled person based upon unfounded assumptions about disability. Graham et al believe that the study 'uncovered the tip of the iceberg of discrimination' (1990: 6).

Sutherland (1981), French et al (1997) and French (1998) talk of more subtle forms of discrimination and prejudice, such as the tendency of potential employers to focus on the supposed incapabilities of disabled people rather than on their capabilities, and demanding that work should be carried out in the same way as non-disabled people perform it. They also discuss at some length the prejudiced attitudes of health and welfare professionals who are unable to accept disabled people as colleagues perhaps because their relationships with disabled people are based on the notion of dependency. French (1988) found that some employers find it particularly difficult to accept disabled people working for or with other disabled people in a professional role. Employers may also ask for abilities which disabled people have had no opportunity to acquire, or ones which are not really needed, such as the ability to drive a car (RADAR 1993, Barnes et al 1998). These are all examples of indirect discrimination. Jolly believes that 'given the overall context it is an achievement that disabled people manage to find work at all' (2000: 801).

Another form of discrimination is the way in which people who become disabled may be given jobs in the same company or place of work which do not reflect their capabilities. Greenwood and Johnson (1987) found that employers tend to focus on semi-skilled and unskilled jobs for disabled people. Jobs may also be reserved for disabled people. In the 1944 Employment Act, for example, the jobs of car park attendant and electrical passenger lift operator were reserved exclusively for disabled people. A similar example of this is the way in which visually impaired people are employed as telephonists by many of the major banks and building societies, in preference to non-disabled people, yet cannot progress up the organisational hierarchy. Deshen (1992), talking of visually impaired telephonists in Israel, mentions the often 'glaring contrast' between the worker's intellectual capacity and his or her job.

Government Schemes and Approaches to the Employment of Disabled People

The major response of government to the employment of disabled people has been one of persuasion aimed at employers. In 1984, for example, the Manpower Services Commission produced its 'Code of Good Practice on the Employment of Disabled People' and in 1990 the Department of Employment introduced its 'two tick' symbol to encourage employers to employ disabled people. They state:

The symbol is a means of publicly showing that your organisation is committed to good policies and practices in the employment of people with disabilities. (1990: 2)

The Government has continued with these campaigns although there is little evidence that they have had any effect (Barnes 1991, Barnes et al 1998). Foley and Pratt state:

The government's continued and exclusive reliance on 'education and persuasion' to overcome the disadvantages faced by disabled people is difficult to understand when its own research so conclusively demonstrates that it has been ineffective in eradicating prejudice and discrimination in employment. (1994: 36)

Special aids, adaptations and services have been available to some disabled employees from government schemes for over 50 years. The Special Aids to Employment Scheme (SAE) was developed in 1944 under the Disabled Person's Employment Act. Disablement Resettlement Officers administered the scheme and later the Disability Advisory Service. These services came together in 1992 to form the Placement, Assessment and Counselling Teams (PACT). The employees of these schemes have always had low status with poor employment prospects and are frequently 'passing through'. These have been cited as reasons for a service that is often inefficient (Roulstone 1998).

Since 1994 the scheme has been subsumed under the Access to Work initiative. Services include adapted computers and an allowance to enable visually impaired employees to pay readers and other assistants. Taxi fares to and from work may also be paid if the disabled person cannot manage or is lacking in public transport or cannot drive. Initially the scheme was entirely financed by government but contributions by employers were set in 1996. This was seen as a retrograde step by many disabled people and their allies. Gooding states that '…by feeding employers assumptions that disabled workers are expensive it will also increase the prejudices faced by all disabled workers' (1994: 5).

Providing disabled people with technology and other services has the potential to widen the range of employment possibilities, as well as the tasks with which they can engage. It has the capacity to remove some access barriers and to enable disabled people to work from home; both of these factors may serve to reduce fatigue and enhance quality of life (Cornes 1991, Roulstone 1998). Technology may also alter perceptions of disabled people, from those of dependency to those of efficiency and independence. This in turn has the potential to shift the meaning of disability from the individual to the environment. As Roulstone states:

The question, what is disability? is opened up for scrutiny when the use of enabling technology provides evidence of once suppressed ability. (1998: 1)

Technology is, however, usually viewed as 'normalising' disabled people and compensating them for their impairments (Oliver 1991). Seale explains that:

> *Microcomputers have been heralded as the new saviours of disabled people because they are believed to have a corrective function, helping disabled people do what they previously could not.* (1998: 260)

Oliver (1990) and Roulstone (1998) contend that little attention has been given to the potential of technology to remove barriers to employment. Issues of technology have been viewed as a technical matter rather than a socio-political matter. Technology is assumed to 'correct' disability which is viewed as residing within the individual. An individual, deficit model of disability has thus been followed which has not been influenced by disabled people themselves (Roulstone 1998). Johnson and Moxon stress the importance of placing technology in context. They state:

> *Of themselves, technologies are neutral; how they are used determines the extent to which they will meet the needs of disabled people. Technology-based services could lead to the greater exclusion of disabled people; alternatively, they could enable people to take increased control of their lives.* (1998: 225)

Access to technology by disabled people is not generally uppermost in the minds of employers which means that when it is introduced there is no guarantee that it will be used in an enabling way (Cornes 1991, Roulstone 1998). Insisting that disabled people can compete on equal terms with non-disabled people by using equipment or other support, can also be a way of denying the extent of disability (French 1994b). The disabled person who uses 'special' equipment may do so, for example, at a much reduced speed. Equipment can also disable people because once it is installed they may be expected to cope without any human assistance or other interventions which can be very difficult and inefficient (French 1991). In addition, as Roulstone (1998) points out, because technology is framed in terms of 'special aids', it inhibits the development and potential of mainstream technology. This, in turn, renders the equipment obscure and expensive which can cause delays in its acquisition and maintenance as well as creating the need for 'special' training.

Employers are unlikely to spend time and money installing technology for people in low status, unstable, or part-time work where disabled people are frequently employed (Burchardt 2000). As Roulstone states 'Social hierarchies profoundly shape access to and use of new technology' (1998: 37). In reality only a minority of disabled people receive such assistance and this depends on the type of work they do, how stable it is, and the severity of their impairments (Roulstone 1998). People in full-time, professional or clerical work are more likely to get help with adaptations as are people with visual impairments (Roulstone 1998). Simkiss et al (1998) found that 85 per cent of the visually impaired employees in their survey received equipment through Access to Work.

The Access to Work initiative can only be used by those already in work or about to start work which means that employers do not have to consider the needs of disabled people until their presence is imminent (Lunt and Thornton 1994) Simkiss et al suggest that a multi-pronged strategy is required to remove employment barriers; they state that 'Behaviour of employers needs to be changed by a combination of compulsion through legislation, persuasion through the business case and through training and ongoing advice and support' (1998: 130).

A recent Government initiative is the New Deal for Disabled People which operates schemes to assist disabled people who have been on long term benefits to find work (The Government's New Deal for Disabled People, RNIB: 1998). This is in response to the Welfare Reform Bill which passed through the House of Commons in June 1999. The New Deal provides training and a personal adviser for four months to assist disabled people into employment (Hermeston 1998). The RNIB is sceptical that the New Deal will be effective unless the Access to Work initiative is strengthened. They recommend a realistic budget that reflects demand; the removal of the employer's contribution; more widely available information to employers; a more coherent service and better training; and an improved career structure for disability employment advisers. Burchardt (2000) believes that inclusion will not be achieved until both impairment-specific and the more general barriers to participation are dismantled.

Equal Opportunities

'Equal opportunities' is not an easy term either to define or to translate into practice. Thompson (1998) believes that equality is an ideological concept and a political term which means different things to different people. Equal opportunity policies have been criticised for their narrow focus on the individual and for their failure to address institutional discrimination (Thompson 1998). They typically concentrate on relatively straightforward matters such as interview practice, recruitment and monitoring the numbers of disabled employees in organisations. Little attempt has been made to organise work so that disabled people can participate in it on an equal level with their peers (Barnes 1991, Farish et al 1995). The restructuring of work, for example to give visually impaired people more time to perform it, or to eliminate the need to drive, is rarely considered (French 1994b). Baron et al (1996) point out that most disabled people, regardless of impairment, need more time to carry out tasks.

The specific needs of disabled people may also be subsumed within a general equal opportunities policy (Barnes et al 1998). Dench et al (1996) found that 48 per cent of the establishments they surveyed had a general policy but only 17 per cent had a specific policy covering disabled people. In their research into social work practice Baron et al found that:

> *All institutions had formal equal opportunity policies, but none made specific reference to issues of disability. Social work staff in the institution were, however, unclear about how the policy was disseminated and put into practice, and felt that it existed in name only. Staff experienced a distinct gap between formal statements of the policy and plans to implement it. In particular staff felt that institutions reacted to specific issues which became defined as 'problems' rather than having a pro-active and comprehensive policy of enabling.* (1996: 368–9)

The idea that the attitude of employers is the most significant barrier to the employment of disabled people, rather than environmental and structural factors, is commonly expressed as is seen in the government's various campaigns of persuasion and in the emphasis on disability awareness training rather than disability equality training (Swain and Lawrence 1994). The notion that disabled people are 'just like everyone else' and therefore need no special help or support is also common. It is stated by the Local Government Management Board that:

> *Most disabled people will not have any special needs and any necessary equipment and assistance can easily be obtained...They share the same hopes and concerns and in most ways will be no different to any other workers you employ.* (1991: 3)

Thompson (1998) believes that equal opportunities does not mean that people from minorities should be treated the same as others but that difference and diversity among people should be promoted. It is, of course, convenient for employers to believe that disabled people want to be treated 'just like everyone else' but disabled people are increasingly demanding the right to be 'equal but different' rather than having to emulate the non-disabled majority (Oliver 1996b).

Farish et al (1995) conducted case studies of colleges and universities in Britain and highlighted how equal opportunity policies for disabled people were not as highly emphasised as those for women or people from ethnic minorities and, where they did exist, were mainly directed at students rather than staff. Financial constraint was frequently cited as a problem and a large gap between rhetoric and practice was usually found.

Equal opportunity policies are overwhelmingly about gender and race with disability being 'tagged on' almost as an afterthought (Baron et al 1996, Hurst 1996). Myers and Parker state that 'During the 1990s it was not uncommon for the discourse of equal opportunities to omit all reference to disabled people' (1996: 66) and Corbett believes that 'equal opportunities' is a 'much abused term' (1996: 22). Equal opportunity policies have done little but raise expectations with minimal result and often exist primarily to present a positive and progressive image of the organisation, to provide 'a smokescreen behind which the status quo remains largely unaffected' (Farish et al 1995: 180).

The Disability Discrimination Act

The Disability Discrimination Act (DDA) was passed in November 1995 on the 14th attempt. The first attempt was made by the deaf MP, Jack Ashley, in 1982. The Act provides the most comprehensive anti-discrimination legislation in Britain to date but does not amount to civil rights legislation though Gooding (1995) describes its introduction as 'a fundamental shift'. There are still many situations where disabled people can be discriminated against legally, many of which are explicitly written into the Act. Cost can be taken into account when deciding whether or not to employ a disabled person as can health and safety regulations. The effect that the disabled person may have on other people, for example customers, can also be put forward as a justification for discrimination (Doyle 1996). The Act is full of loopholes and phrases such as 'if it is reasonable' as well as vague and ill-defined words such as 'substantial'. It is nowhere near as robust as the Sex Discrimination Act (1975) and the Race Relations Act (1976) and has been dubbed the 'Doesn't Do Anything Act' by disabled people themselves (Trade Union Disability Alliance 1997). Full human and civil rights legislation for disabled people is in place in other parts of the world including the USA, Sweden, New Zealand and Australia (Cooper and Vernon 1996).

Disability is defined in terms of impairment which is, in turn, defined very narrowly. The guiding principle is the severity of the impairment rather than the degree of discrimination experienced. The right to fair treatment is, therefore, rationed. Drug addiction is not covered by the Act and nor is being HIV positive until symptoms are apparent. Mental health problems are included in the Act provided they are 'clinically well recognised'. There is no guarantee that a person who is classified as disabled under another classification system will be classified as disabled under the DDA. Because disability is individualised, institutional discrimination and indirect discrimination are barely recognised.

The DDA gives disabled people rights in the following areas:

- Employment.
- The provision of goods, facilities and services.
- Buying and renting land and property.

The Act can be seen to be piecemeal legislation as large areas of life, such as education and transport, are not included or are only included to a very limited extent. All that colleges are required to do, for example, is to provide a statement of intent with regard to disabled students. New transport has to meet minimum standards for disabled people but this only applies to land-based transport.

Even those areas which are covered by the Act are full of loop-holes and exemptions. With regard to employment, the Act only applies if more that 15 people are employed. The Act does not apply to some types of employment, such as the fire, prison and police services, and employers are under no obligation to make their work places accessible until a disabled person is in post. Gooding states:

> *There is no general duty on employers to act pro-actively so as to make their work places more accessible to disabled employees. Instead, the duty to make reasonable adjustments is owed to individual disabled persons when the relevant circumstances arise.* (1996: 20)

It is, therefore, legal to discriminate against disabled people in many areas of life and discrimination can be justified, for example by employers, in a way that it cannot be justified in the Sex Discrimination Act (1975) and the Race Relations Act (1976). Positive discrimination in favour of disabled people is not required by the Act but is not unlawful.

Reasonable adjustments to employment, as stated in the Act, could be very beneficial to disabled people if they were enforced. They include:

- Making adjustments to premises.
- Allocating some of the disabled person's duties to another person.
- Transferring a disabled person to an existing vacancy.
- Altering working hours.
- Assigning a disabled person to a different place of work.
- Allowing time off work for rehabilitation, assessment and treatment.
- Giving and arranging training.
- Modifying or acquiring equipment.
- Modifying instructions or reference manuals.
- Modifying procedures for testing or assessment.
- Providing a reader or interpreter.
- Providing supervision.

A major limitation of the Act, until April 2000, was that there was no commission, that is no body to take up people's complaints. Disabled people had to launch their own complaints which were conducted mainly through industrial tribunals rather than the courts. The Disability Rights Commission is, however, now in place. It remains to be seen how helpful it will be as it will operate within the restraints of very weak legislation. This has led many people to believe that the Act should be scrapped and reformulated because it is so fundamentally flawed (Trade Union Disability Alliance 1997). The Rights Now Campaign, which is a coalition of organisations of and for disabled people, as well as other organisation such as the Trade Union Congress (TUC) and Liberty, are campaigning to bring about fully comprehensive disability discrimination legislation. The passing of comprehensive disability discrimination legislation is a major goal and area of activity of the disabled people's movement. The campaign is likely to continue until civil rights legislation, similar to that for women and people from ethnic minorities, becomes a reality.

The major reasons put forward over the years for failing to pass fully comprehensive disability discrimination legislation are firstly that disabled people are all so different that no meaningful changes can be made, and secondly that such legislation would be too expensive. The first reflects a defeatist attitude that focuses on impairment rather than the commonalities of disability, and the second may be considered flawed because, if the environment were to be made more accessible to disabled people, they could be an economic asset. This was, indeed, a major argument for getting disability discrimination legislation on to the statute books in the USA (Foley and Pratt 1994). Oliver states:

> *Protagonists argue that the Act will pay for itself in that by reducing employment discrimination, it will both raise tax revenues and reduce welfare payments. Further, opening up access to goods and services to disabled people will stimulate new demands in the economy.* (1996b: 117)

The success of the Act will also depends on how far it is enforced. As noted above, the quota scheme, introduced in 1944, was ineffective. The new legislation does, however, demand, albeit in a limited way, the removal of barriers to employment for some disabled people.

In October 2000 the 1998 Human Rights Act came into effect in Britain. This Act incorporates the rights contained within the European Convention on Human Rights into British law. These rights include:

- The right to privacy and family life.
- The right to marry and found a family.
- The right to education.

Most of these rights are, however, qualified and can be infringed in certain circumstances. Public authorities have a duty to comply with the Act bur private companies and individuals do not have any obligations under the Act unless any of their functions are public.

The Human Rights Act may, in some circumstances, enhance the DDA. The right to education, for example, may be used to address some of the issues faced by disabled children and students, and the right to marry and found a family may be used to address issues pertaining to institutional living. In addition, what is considered 'reasonable' by the courts under the DDA, will have to take the Human Rights Act into account (Casserley 2000).

The Employment of Visually Impaired People

In 1991 the RNIB published the first nation-wide survey of visually impaired adults in Britain (Bruce et al 1991). The survey was conducted between November 1986 and April 1987 and was designed to complement the OPCS government surveys of disabled people. Structured interviews were conducted with 595 visually impaired people who were registered or eligible for registration as blind or partially sighted. The areas covered included leisure, mobility, education, reading habits, and employment. The survey was limited to visually impaired people of 16 years and over who were living in private households.

The survey revealed that only 25 per cent of visually impaired people of working age (from 16 to 64 for men, and 16 to 59 for women) were in full or part-time paid employment. Of these 75 per cent were doing the same job as they were before the onset of visual impairment. The figure of 25 per cent represents 22,000 employed visually impaired people (RNIB 1996a). The total number of visually impaired people in full or part-time employment is, however, 30,000 as 8,000 people continue to work beyond retirement age (Bruce et al 1991).

Seventeen per cent of blind people, and 31 per cent of partially sighted people were working. This compared with a 31 per cent employment rate for disabled people overall at that time (Martin et al 1988). Bruce et al state that '...not being in paid employment is normal for visually impaired people of working age' (1991: 235). This is despite the fact that visually impaired graduates gain the same level of qualifications as sighted graduates (RNIB 1996b, Simkiss et al 1998).

A survey carried out by Simkiss et al (1998) of 172 visually impaired people was, however, more optimistic. They found that 32 per cent of those of working age were employed and, of those who had been through higher education, 40 per cent were employed compared with 17 per cent who had not.

Tillsley (1997) found that half of those in his survey with partial sight were working compared with one in six of those who were blind, and that those with the highest qualifications were the most successful in finding employment. Sixty nine per cent of visually impaired people reported leaving their work because of disability or injury, and 88 per cent had been out of work for a year compared with 73 per cent of other disabled people and 47 per cent of the general population (Bruce et al 1991). Most unemployed visually impaired people lose their jobs within six months of the onset of visual impairment (RNIB 1996a).

Wide scale unemployment is likely to foster a particular image of visually impaired people. As Apter states:

Unemployment of people with severe visual disabilities is a major factor in society's perception of the capabilities, independence, and social participation of these individuals. (1992: 22)

Winyard (1996) found that the unemployment rate among visually disabled people was two and a half times the national average and Dench et al (1996) found that over half of the employers they surveyed said that they would not employ someone who had 'difficulty in seeing'. Curtis et al believe that:

There is a deep rooted prejudice and ignorance by many employers and employees as to the ability of visually impaired people to function effectively in the work place. (1997: 18)

A sizeable minority of visually impaired people of working age have additional impairments which may further impede their employment chances. Simkiss et al (1998) found that 26 per cent of their sample reported an additional impairment or illness. With visually impaired children this figure rises to 56 per cent (Walker et al 1992). Barnes et al (1998) and Burchardt (2000) confirm that the more severe the overall level of impairment the more difficult it is to find work and that the severity of the impairment is more significant than the type of impairment.

Visually impaired people are less likely to be in professional jobs than non-disabled or disabled people generally as Table 2.1 illustrates.

Simkiss et al (1998), however, report that 29 per cent of their sample of visually impaired employees were in professional posts. This sample was, however, taken from people who had contacted the RNIB Student Support Service, thus a high proportion would have undertaken further and higher education.

Thirteen per cent of visually impaired people of working age are self-employed compared with ten per cent of the general population (Bruce et al

Table 2.1 Occupational status of visually impaired people, disabled people and non-disabled people

	Professional	Semi-skilled and unskilled
Visually impaired people	14%	36%
Disabled people	25%	31%
Non-disabled people	34%	23%

Source: Adapted from Bruce, I., McKennell, A. and Walker, E. (1991), *Blind and Partially Sighted Adults in Britain: The RNIB Survey*, HMSO Publications, London.

1991). This may indicate the inhospitable nature of the work environment for visually impaired people. As Deshen states 'The situation of self-employment has the potential for obviating the pain of the social ramifications of blindness' (1992: 72). Sly (1996) found that disabled people are slightly more likely to be self-employed than non-disabled people with over two thirds of the self-employed being men. Similar findings are reported by Burchardt (2000). Many chose self-employment for reasons related to disability. Barnes et al (1998) point out that self-employed people tend to work longer hours and are among those with the lowest pay.

Table 2.2 shows that nearly half of those who do find new employment following the onset of visual impairment, experience a lowering of occupational status, although 25 per cent find work of a higher status.

Visually impaired people in professional occupations comprise 14 per cent of the 22,000 visually impaired people in employment, that is approximately 3080 people. It is estimated that there are approximately 250 visually impaired physiotherapists practising in Britain which comprises about eight per cent of visually impaired people in professional occupations.

Table 2.2 Occupational status following the onset of visual impairment

The same status	32%
Lower status	43%
Higher status	25%

Source: Adapted from Bruce, I., McKennell, A. and Walker, E. (1991), *Blind and Partially Sighted Adults in Britain: The RNIB Survey*, HMSO Publications, London.

Conclusion

This chapter has highlighted the situation of disabled people, including visually impaired people, in the employment market in Britain. Barnes et al (1998) point out, however, that there are enormous gaps in the research, including the employment situation of disabled people from ethnic minorities and the experiences of disabled people themselves. It is hoped that the study of visually impaired physiotherapists presented in Part Two of this book will give voice to one particular group of disabled employees and that this will be relevant to other disabled employees.

Many of the issues raised in this chapter will be re-visited in the analysis of the experiences of the visually impaired physiotherapists. These will include barriers to post-registration education, the effects of technology, the effects of government schemes and legislation, and the attitudes and behaviour of employers, colleagues and the Chartered Society of Physiotherapy. The following chapter will review the literature on the attitudes of health and welfare professionals towards disabled people and the experiences of disabled people who work within the health and welfare professions including doctors, social workers and prosthetists. This will provide further contextual information for analysing the employment experiences of visually impaired physiotherapists.

Chapter 3

Disabled Health and Welfare Professionals

The first part of this chapter presents a general overview of the attitudes of health and welfare professionals towards disabled people and, in particular, their attitudes towards the recruitment of disabled people as their colleagues. The second part of the chapter focuses on the experiences of disabled health and welfare professionals.

Attitudes of Health and Welfare Professionals Towards the Recruitment of Disabled Colleagues

Disabled people are widely discriminated against in most types of employment (Barnes et al 1998, Burchardt 2000) which makes it likely that they will find entry to employment of professional status, such as the health and welfare professions, particularly difficult. It was noted in chapter 2 that disabled people are under-represented in professional employment. Although it might be considered that health and welfare professionals would be particularly knowledgeable and understanding regarding disabled people, there is considerable evidence to suggest that they have not been especially positive in their attitudes or knowledgeable about the implications of disability (Abberley 1995, French 1997a). Baron et al talking of social workers state:

> Most of the practice teachers admitted they had given little forethought on the suitability of their working environment to disabled colleagues and only did so when asked to take on a disabled student. (1996: 367)

Although attitudes may have improved in recent years, with, for example, the introduction of 'equal opportunity' policies and the Disability Discrimination Act (1995), the career literature of the CSP, which was published in 1984, states:

> Any form of physical disability or weakness is likely to contra-indicate physiotherapy as a suitable career, in particular defects in hearing, epilepsy, chest

ailments, skin conditions, heart defects, nervous breakdowns. Injuries to backs, knees and hands may also prejudice acceptance for training. (1984: 2)

Although an exception is made for visually impaired candidates entering the physiotherapy profession, because of their historical connection with the profession over the course of this century and their own 'special' college (see chapter 4), they too were expected to be fit and free of any other impairments. In the prospectus of the North London School of Physiotherapy for the Visually Handicapped (formally the RNIB School of Physiotherapy) it is stated that 'Physiotherapy is an unsuitable career choice if you have any mental or physical disability or sensory impairment other than visual impairment' (1990: 2).

The 1998 career literature of the CSP shows a distinct change of policy towards disabled candidates and other minority groups. Some of the responsibility for the inclusion of visually impaired students in mainstream colleges is, however, focused on the RNIB and it is clear that disability is viewed within the perspective of the individual model:

The Chartered Society of Physiotherapy, and the courses it approves, work towards equal opportunities of access. They welcome applicants regardless of sex, age, race, ethnic or national origin, sexual orientation, social class, family responsibilities, political and religious beliefs...Students with a visual impairment can now train on mainstream physiotherapy programmes with support from the Royal National Institute for the Blind. Students are advised to discuss ways of getting on to the course and the specific support required with the RNIB Physiotherapy Support Manager...Sympathetic consideration is given to applicants who have a physical disability including a careful assessment of the extent of their disability to ensure that they can meet the demands of the course. (1998: 10)

Attitudes and behaviour towards disabled people in other health professions have also tended to be mixed. Moon (1990) carried out a study of 12 nurses who became disabled, only four of whom were still employed. She found their experiences very variable but overall the help they received was inadequate and patchy. There was disagreement between the disabled nurses and their employers in 50 per cent of cases about whether the impairment would affect their ability to work.

Goffman (1968) wrote about disabled people having a discredited social identity whereby disability becomes their 'master status' obscuring all other attributes. He believed that those who associated closely with disabled people on an equal basis were likely to acquire a 'courtesy stigma' whereby they became 'contaminated' themselves. This perceived spoiling of image may be a further reason why disabled people are not accepted in the health and welfare professions in greater numbers.

The need for effective social interaction and good communication skills is strongly emphasised by many of the health and welfare professions (French 1986), and the belief that disabled people lack these skills may serve as a powerful justification for their exclusion. Edwards (1986), a blind speech and language pathology student, was told by staff that a blind person would be a poor model of communication for sighted people, and was criticised for not making eye contact with clients which, despite her blindness, was thought to be deliberate. Several visually impaired health and welfare professionals interviewed by French (1986) had similar experiences. In contrast, disabled people may be perceived as having more insight or greater perception than others (French 1995) though there is no evidence of difference in many cognitive and sensory abilities (Lewis 1987).

In a questionnaire study French (1987) found that the attitudes of physiotherapists towards hypothetical people with various impairments, appeared to be similar to those of the general public; for example when asked which people would be suitable candidates for physiotherapy education, 95 per cent (198) were in favour of recruiting people with controlled diabetes, but only 61 per cent (127) were in favour of recruiting people with controlled epilepsy. Thirty three per cent (69) thought people who had experienced clinical depression or anxiety in the past were unsuitable candidates for physiotherapy.

Elliott et al (1992) found that occupational therapists generally have favourable attitudes towards disabled colleagues with the exception of those diagnosed with drug dependency and psychiatric disorders. The number of years the person had been practising occupational therapy, and the quality or quantity of contact with disabled people, made no difference to their assessment of disabled colleagues. Colorez and Geist (1987) found little difference between general employers and rehabilitation employers regarding attitudes about recruiting disabled workers and, in a review of the literature, French (1997d) found little evidence of difference between the attitudes of health and welfare professionals towards disabled people and the attitudes of the general public although the research findings, which were derived from many different methodologies, did conflict. Scullion (1999) found, in his study of the attitudes of student nurses and their teachers, that '...there is little interest in disability other than as a medicalised phenomenon...disability has little recognition by nurses as a social issue' (1999: 554). Allen and Birse state:

Health care professionals share the values and expectations of their society and show the same reactions that unstigmatised individuals have towards those with differences. (1991: 150)

Most of the overt justification for the exclusion of disabled people from the health and welfare professions is in terms of the disabled people themselves; their presumed inability to cope, the adverse effect they may have on patients and clients, and the assumption of proneness to accidents (Libman 1985, French 1995). Negative attitudes are sometimes rationalised and disguised as concern, emphasising that disabled people may damage themselves or others, by undertaking such demanding work. Edwards states:

> *Another time I was working with a pre-school aged child, playing on the floor. My supervisor again took me aside following the session and told me that I should not do therapy on the floor since the child's toys would be left around and I would fall down and hurt myself and possibly the child.* (1986: 309)

It is even possible that the views of health and welfare professionals are more negative than those of the general public due to the unequal relationship they have with disabled people, and the fact that they come into contact only when disabled people are deemed to need their help (Gething 1993).

Sociologists and disabled people have commented on the paternalism of medical practice (Hugman 1991, Davis 1993b, Finkelstein and Stuart 1996, Oliver 1996b). Sutherland (1981) notes that professionals base their dealings on a dependency model in which they are the experts and disabled people are dependent on them for help. When discussing the issue of disabled people becoming health professionals he states, 'Since the job for which the person is applying would confer a recognition of equality, they tend not to get it, they are judged unsuitable' (1981: 40). Chinnery (1991) points out that there are few disabled people employed in the health and welfare services in Britain and that most of those who are employed manage to 'pass' as non-disabled.

There is evidence to suggest that disability may be just one attribute which is considered undesirable in members of the health and welfare professions; race and class discrimination, for example, are well documented (Fernando 1989, CSP 1996). In the case of the physiotherapy profession, gender discrimination has been in favour of women until recent times when men have been particularly welcomed (Barclay 1994). Men are, however, disproportionately and favourably represented in senior management and academic posts (CSP 1996). In addition French (1987) found that various characteristics which go against the stereotyped image of the physiotherapist are stigmatised by that profession; for example, to be very over weight was considered more of a barrier to recruitment than blindness or using a wheelchair. The social acceptability of an impairment may, therefore, be more important than the limitations to which it may give rise.

A further factor which may exclude disabled people from the health and welfare professions is that of social class (Preece 1996). Although the situation has improved, health and welfare professionals tend to come from middle-class backgrounds whereas the majority of disabled people come from working class homes (Jacobson et al 1991). Goffman (1969) suggested that in order to maintain their status and power, professionals need to keep a certain distance between themselves and their clients, thus professional members of less power and status may be perceived as a threat because they lessen that distance. Drawing upon his dramaturgical model, where he perceives social life as akin to theatre, he states, 'If the team is to maintain the impression that it is fostering then there must be some assurance that no individual will be allowed to join both team and audience' (1969: 97). Yet by definition a disabled health or welfare professional would belong to both groups.

Sutherland believes that the stigma of low socio-economic class is added to that of disability and, conversely, that a middle class background may serve to reduce the stigma of disability. He explains:

It is much easier to counteract the stereotyped ideas about disability on which discrimination is based if one possesses a middle-class background and accent, a university education and the particular type of articulacy and confidence that these factors produce. (1981: 35)

It is unclear whether disabled people are actively discouraged from entering the health and welfare professions, but it seems likely that the acceptance of more than a few could seriously challenge the traditional professional/client relationship where the professional is considered to be the expert and occupies a dominant position over the patient or client. Sociologists and disabled people alike have written extensively of the conflicts in the professional/client relationship which often seem to arise through differing conceptions and definitions of illness and disability (Hugman 1991, French 1997a). Disabled people are likely to possess skills which non-disabled professionals lack, yet in order to improve their skills professionals need to learn from their disabled clients which, in turn, could lead to a reduction in their own authority and status (Finkelstein and Stuart 1996, French et al 1997).

In a content analysis of the career literature of 26 health and welfare professions and occupations, French (1986) found that disabled people were never specifically invited to apply, yet ten of these professions and occupations specifically sought candidates with the ability to empathise and understand ill and disabled people. The radiography profession, for example, was seeking people having tact and empathy (College of Radiographers 1985) and the audiology technician was required to have 'a sympathetic and understanding personality' (British Society of Audiology, undated). These are qualities which disabled people, by virtue of their experience, are, perhaps, more likely to possess. Burnfield, a psychiatrist with multiple sclerosis, states:

> *I believe that having MS has helped me to become more sensitive to the needs of others and that it has enhanced my skills as a healer. I often think of myself as being doubly qualified, firstly as a patient and secondly as a doctor – the order is important.* (1985: 169)

There is an ancient maxim that 'only the wounded physician heals' (Bennet 1987: 206); it is a common belief that the only way to gain full understanding of any event or situation is to experience it oneself. Stetten (1983), a visually impaired physician, claims to have learned far more about visual impairment from chance contact with other visually impaired people than from ophthalmologists whom, he believes, confine their real interest in medicine 'to events which occur within the globe of the eye' (1983: 27). This impression is confirmed by Parrish, an ophthalmologist, who refers to blindness as 'our ultimate professional failure' (1988: 31). In the 1980s and 1990s there has been a huge expansion of self-help groups which are often based around notions of mutual understanding and assistance.

Turner is of the opinion that excluding disabled people from the health and welfare professions is nothing short of hypocrisy. He states:

> *How can we tell patients they can lead normal lives when we don't allow their peers to become our colleagues? Though not yet illegal to discriminate on health grounds, there can be no doubt that it is immoral and unethical to do so.* (1984: 451)

It should be remembered, however, that the views put forward by professional bodies do not necessarily reflect the views of their membership. Many health and welfare professionals agree that disabled people may have unique assets to offer these professions inasmuch as their personal experience of disability, and their identification with disabled patients and clients, gives them a dimension of knowledge that others may not share (Turner 1984, Teager 1987). Craik (1990) asserts that the profession of occupational therapy welcomes disabled applicants and that their numbers are increasing, and studies carried out by the American Society of Handicapped Physicians show that approximately 75 per cent of doctors, with a wide variety of impairments, remain successfully employed in clinical practice (Wainapel and Bernbaum 1986).

Perceptions and Experiences of Disabled Health and Welfare Professionals

There has been very little research specifically addressing the perceptions and experiences of disabled health and welfare professionals. Because of the paucity of research in this area, the rest of this chapter will examine a small study of 25 health and welfare professionals, who were accepted for professional education despite substantial impairments (French 1986, 1988). The aim of this research was to discover their experiences both during training and when qualified. The issues raised were wide-ranging and included the attitudes and behaviour of college lecturers, colleagues and patients and clients; the possible advantages of disability within their professional role; the problems experienced in training and employment; and whether they found it safe to reveal their impairments.

The study was based upon semi-structured interviews with 25 disabled people who were employed or training in the health and welfare professions. The sample consisted of nine men and 16 women and represented seven professions and 17 types of impairment; two people had dual qualifications. All but two of the research respondents were accepted for professional education as disabled people, the others acquired their impairments during training.

Perceived Advantages and Disadvantages of being a Disabled Health or Welfare Professional

All the disabled professionals could see advantages relating to being disabled in the work context. The most common response was that they felt better able to empathise with their patients and clients and understand the social and psychological implications of disability. Most felt they could empathise with and understand those with a similar impairment best. A hearing impaired therapist said:

> I've got a lot more patience with deaf people and I get more out of them. The doctors say 'forget it, ask a relative' but I speak to them.

All the deaf people found the ability to lip read helpful. One mentioned her skill at communicating with patients with tracheostomies, and another found she could lip read patients when nobody else could understand them. One spoke sign language fluently and was sometimes used as an interpreter.

Most of the disabled professionals believed they had more knowledge of disability, and a different type of knowledge, than their colleagues. A prosthetist who had a lower limb amputation himself stated:

They (patients) want to pick your brain for every bit of knowledge they can get. They're very interested to find out how you coped.

He found he was able to identify patients' problems, especially the small, less obvious ones which other prosthetists might miss or regard as trivial.

Some reported that their patients and clients frequently commented on the advantage of the professional's disability from their own point of view. A prosthetist with an amputation himself remarked 'Patients say, 'you've got one, you know what I mean'. Similarly a doctor said:

Very many people have told me they can talk to me because I know what it feels like to have an illness. Once you get over that hump of being accepted (for training) then you can use your disability.

Others spoke of the advantage of needing help from their patients and clients. A counsellor explained, 'By me needing help it's actually saying 'This is a partnership''. Similarly a blind social worker commented:

I'm able to say to my clients, 'I'll help you but there are certain ways in which you are going to have to help me', and the client doesn't feel totally taken over or totally worthless.

Some people felt that the advantages of being disabled not only cancelled out any disadvantages there might be but actually outweighed them. A doctor commented:

MS has been something I've used. Having MS has been an added dimension in my training, in my understanding of people, and in the development of my expertise and skills.

And a prosthetist said:

You have a great understanding of their problems because no matter how good a prosthetist is, if he's got two legs he falls short of really knowing what it's like.

However, two of the disabled professionals firmly believed that being disabled gave them no additional insight into disability, and one person with a congenital impairment said she had no special understanding of acquired impairment.

Some people pointed out the advantages of their work from a personal point of view. Several physically impaired physiotherapists mentioned that the active nature of the job benefited them physically, and a number of people with sensory impairments believed the nature of the work prevented them from becoming isolated. A deaf therapist said 'I do feel that if I didn't have this type of job, where I'm meeting different people every day, I would withdraw very quickly into myself'.

A few of the disabled professionals pointed out the disadvantages that could arise as a result of being disabled when interacting with patients or clients. A doctor felt that his severe impairment inhibited patients with mental health problems from discussing their difficulties, and a psychiatrist found that some of his patients had a tendency to mother him and could find it difficult in psychoanalysis to express anger or hostility for fear that it would damage him in some way. An occupational therapist found that elderly, confused patients and clients occasionally lacked confidence in her but she managed the situation by reassuring them and immediately focusing attention back on them.

A blind social worker found lack of non-verbal communication a problem, though others felt able to compensate and even viewed blindness as helpful in some situations. For example, a social worker felt that clients could speak more honestly to him because they knew he could not recognise them in other contexts, and a counsellor reported that clients found her blindness helped them to speak more openly. A prosthetist with an amputation himself noted that patients could be discouraged by seeing him cope so well. They would sometimes say, 'If only I could walk like you'. He was, however, acutely aware of this and was very careful never to compare himself with his clients.

Access to Professional Education

Of the 23 disabled professionals who had been accepted for professional education as disabled people, eight reported that their entry qualifications were higher than average, and five thought that this was a major factor in their acceptance for professional education. A further eight said that they had been helped to gain access to professional education by an influential person. Such people were either doctors of high status who knew the individual personally, or someone on the selection panel with particular knowledge or interest in disability; for example a person interviewing a blind candidate had a visually impaired son. Twelve people felt that their acceptance for professional education had been strongly influenced by one of these two factors. In addition a doctor mentioned the advantage of his socially privileged background, and several people indicated that they came from 'medical' families.

All but one person revealed their impairments before the selection interview. Several, especially those with relatively hidden impairments, were uncertain of the wisdom of this and spoke of being in a dilemma. A profoundly deaf person felt it was best to reveal her disability after contact had been made because of the 'funny ideas' people have about deafness.

Some of the disabled people interviewed by Duckett also chose not to reveal their impairments. One person said:

> *Putting epilepsy down on the application form is the same as asking the employer to put your application in the bin. If you are going to do that you might as well bin your application yourself and cut out the middleman.* (2000: 1030)

Of the 23 health and welfare professionals who were accepted for professional education as disabled people, eight experienced difficulty. An occupational therapist stated, 'It didn't matter what I said, they said I couldn't cope', and a physiotherapist recalled, 'His parting words were 'nobody will accept you as a physio, no school's going to accept you''. Interestingly she was later accepted by the very person who had said this. Several people mentioned that getting as far as the interview was the main problem, a counsellor concluded that professionals 'have conditioned themselves to believing that the disabled person is the person who should be helped rather than the helper'.

Some people were turned down by one college on the grounds of disability, but were willingly accepted by another. Several people who were refused entry to physiotherapy education because of disability gained access to occupational therapy without difficulty, and one person who was told by her school career service that every type of work involving patients would be out of the question, was accepted into pharmacy, nursing, and physiotherapy. It must be emphasised, however, that the majority of the disabled professionals, 15 of the 23, experienced no problems regarding their acceptance for professional education.

Attitudes and Behaviour of Teachers

Some people experienced negative attitudes and behaviour from their teachers. The most common complaint was a general lack of adaptation to meet their needs. A physiotherapist recalled 'They weren't obstructive, but they didn't go out of their way to be helpful either', and a deaf therapist said 'I couldn't follow the lectures at all, yet I didn't feel I could keep saying 'I'm deaf, will you look at me?''. Some felt they were viewed in terms of being disabled, while others mentioned that their teachers lacked confidence in them. Several blind people complained of the excessive concern over their inability to make eye contact with patients and clients and the difficulty they had convincing teaching staff that they could cope.

A doctor who acquired his impairment during training felt unable to confide in the staff. He explained:

> *I was very frightened that if I had a disease like that they might suggest that I wasn't able to continue the training and that I wouldn't qualify. I felt if I mentioned them (the symptoms) they'd think I was skiving, or malingering or being a hypochondriac or neurotic, and I wasn't going to be labelled as those things.*

Similarly, a physiotherapist said 'I had to try and keep a brave face on it and not let on, I thought it might affect my career, they might just chuck me out'.

Twelve of the disabled professionals could recall negative attitudes and behaviour from their teachers, although they all related instances of positive attitudes and behaviour too. The remaining 13 regarded the attitudes and behaviour of their teachers as either neutral or good. A physiotherapist said that she could not recall 'any aggravation at any level', and an occupational therapist stated 'It didn't matter what problems I had, I just had to go to them and they'd say 'OK, there's a way round it''. Despite the various difficulties experienced, only six people failed to complete their courses in the minimum possible time.

Employment

The attitudes and behaviour of colleagues were reported as being overwhelmingly good, although a few people mentioned a certain lack of understanding saying that their colleagues tended to forget or deny that they were disabled which could create difficulties. A deaf therapist, for example, said that people forgot to look at her when speaking, and a blind social worker said that certain colleagues felt snubbed when he did not respond to their smiles and waves. Some people said they had really to press for what they needed. A visually impaired social worker, for example, had to fight for an office where he could adjust the lighting and get away from colleagues who were so fascinated by his specialised equipment that he could not get on with his work. Several people said that colleagues failed to realise that to produce the same quantity and quality of work, it was necessary to work both harder and longer.

Both during their education and after qualifying some people said they had been encouraged by senior colleagues to work with disabled people, or in areas of medicine considered to be of low prestige. A blind person was accepted for a post on the condition that initially he would work with blind clients. A counsellor commented, 'They always assumed I'd do disability counselling, they were hanging a label round my neck'. A physiotherapist was asked, 'Don't you think you should be working with the young chronic sick?' and an occupational therapist was advised to work in psychiatry. After successfully qualifying, two people were advised by members of their own profession to do full time voluntary work. Some people decided to work with those with the same type of impairment as themselves. This could lead to suspicion; two people complained that colleagues thought they might 'over-identify' thereby lacking 'objectivity'.

Most people, however, had met with positive attitudes and behaviour at work. A deaf therapist commented, 'I depend a little on the staff but they never seem to mind, they never force me into anything'. Only three people reported any instances of negative attitudes or behaviour from patients or clients.

Just four of the disabled professionals had difficulty finding work. However, a few did meet with negative attitudes in the process. At her first interview in a large London teaching hospital, an occupational therapist was told, 'I must be perfectly honest, I don't see any point in showing you round'. One problem encountered was the expectation in some of these professions that newly qualified staff should 'rotate' to different medical specialities thereby gaining varied experience, a practice not possible for all the disabled professionals. Some people observed that working in senior posts was easier. A deaf occupational therapist spoke extensively of the advantages of being in charge. She explained 'I'm the boss and I delegate what I can't do. I'm in control and I know what's going on, all communication comes through me'.

Some people felt that in order to cope, both during professional education and at work, it was necessary to work harder and be more determined, they spoke of a need to 'prove' themselves. Others had come to the conclusion, however, that these feelings originated, at least in part, from within themselves; a blind person had started to ask himself 'To whom am I proving what?'.

Where possible people tended to specialise early. They tried to find work where they could function well, for example a deaf person said she would avoid a position which involved treating patients or clients in groups, and would never work in a very large hospital. However, people with the same type of impairment had differing views concerning the suitability or unsuitability of various areas of work; this seemed to be due to the severity of the impairment, to personality factors and to the particular work settings they were in.

Fifteen of the disabled professionals were restricted in the type of work they could do. For example a doctor who used crutches said he would find surgery difficult and could not visit patients at home because of access problems. However, by choosing their specialities and places of work carefully, most people reported that they could fulfil all of their work obligations.

The findings of this small study show that the majority of the disabled professionals had received positive treatment from teachers and colleagues during their professional education and careers. A sizeable minority, however, had experienced some degree of negative discrimination either as a result of work practices and structures or their colleagues' and teachers' behaviour and lack of understanding. Most of these problems occurred when attempting to gain access to, and during professional education. At this stage disabled individuals have no professional status themselves which may serve to reduce the negative perceptions of disability when they qualify. The inequalities inherent in the teacher/student relationship may also create a situation where negative attitudes and behaviour can be expressed more readily, especially as the educational structures of many of these professions have, until recently, been highly authoritarian. This small study suggests that disabled professionals are no less capable than their non-disabled colleagues and that they may have unique assets to bring to these professions.

Conclusion

This chapter has explored the attitudes and behaviour of health and welfare professionals towards disabled people and the experiences of a small sample of disabled health and welfare professionals. This will serve as a back-drop to compare, contrast and analyse the experiences of the visually impaired physiotherapists. It will provide an opportunity to compare the situation of visually impaired physiotherapists with other visually impaired health and welfare professionals as well as those with other impairments.

PART 2

THE EXPERIENCES OF VISUALLY IMPAIRED PHYSIOTHERAPISTS

Chapter 4

Visually Impaired Physiotherapists: An Historical Overview

This chapter will provide an historical overview of the physiotherapy profession over the course of the 20th century focusing in particular on visually impaired physiotherapists. It will highlight some of the major changes which have taken place within the physiotherapy profession as well as wider changes such as the effects of the First and Second World Wars on health care, and the introduction of the NHS. The chapter will examine some of the difficulties visually impaired physiotherapists have experienced over the course of this century and how their place within the profession has been maintained.

Physiotherapy arose from the profession of nursing at the end of the 19th century, although many of its treatment techniques, such as manipulation, massage, and hydrotherapy were used by the Ancient Romans and Greeks. The physiotherapy profession was founded by four nurses and midwives who were all trained in 'medical rubbing' (Barclay 1994). They established the Society of Trained Masseuses (STM) in 1894, which changed its name to the Incorporated Society of Trained Masseuses (ISTM) in 1900 following registration with the Board of Trade.

Members of ISTM were referred to as masseuses and masseurs but later became known as physiotherapists; the early membership consisted entirely of women. Candidates were initially examined in massage, but in 1910 an examination in remedial exercises was introduced, and in 1915 an examination in medical electricity was added (Thornton 1994). Training in the early days was carried out by means of private tuition. In 1920 the Society was granted a Royal Charter and changed its name to the Chartered Society of Massage and Remedial Gymnastics. Its name was changed again in 1942 to the Chartered Society of Physiotherapy.

Visually Impaired Physiotherapists

Reference was made to blind masseuses as early as 1891 in the Minute Book of the British and Foreign Blind Association (the forerunner of the RNIB) where it was proposed that two blind girls would be taught massage (Thomas

1957). It is estimated that by the early 1900s there were approximately 50 certified blind masseuses and masseurs practising in Britain (St. Dunstan's. Undated). The existence of visually impaired people in this area of work was not, however, new; in Japan visually impaired people had had the exclusive right to practise massage for hundreds of years (Yoshimoto 1901).

The British and Foreign Blind Association became the National Institute for the Blind (NIB) in 1914, changing its name to the Royal National Institute for the Blind (RNIB) in 1953 following the granting of a Royal Charter in 1948. The institute has supported the training of visually impaired physiotherapists from the First World War to the present day. Until 1995 it administered its own School of Physiotherapy for visually impaired students in London. By 1987 more than 900 visually impaired students, many from overseas, had trained as physiotherapists through the RNIB, and approximately 400 were working throughout the world (Teager 1987). About 200 of these physiotherapists were ex-service men who were blinded in action (RNIB Undated).

The School of Physiotherapy underwent several changes of name throughout its history. In 1944 it changed from the NIB School of Massage and Electrotherapy, to the NIB School of Physiotherapy. In 1953 it changed its name to the RNIB School of Physiotherapy. This name remained until 1978 when the school moved to new premises in Highgate when it changed to The North London School of Physiotherapy for the Visually Handicapped (NLSP).

The first visually impaired students were formally trained in massage in the United Kingdom in 1895 at the Henshaw's Blind Asylum in Manchester; their skills were examined by the asylum's physician. It is stated:

> Your board arranged with Mrs. Abernethy Rose to teach the massage treatment to three girls...Dr. Jones, physician to the asylum, has certified that they are proficient masseurs... When it is known that the asylum can supply good operators, no difficulty will be experienced in finding employment for them.
> (Henshaw's Blind Asylum 1895: 7)

Training under Dr. Fletcher Little

In 1900 visually impaired students were integrated with sighted students at the London School of Massage in London which was run by Dr. Fletcher Little. The students underwent a three to six month training at the end of which Dr. Fletcher Little conducted an examination and issued his own certificates. He recognised the potential of visually impaired people, although he would only accept the most able. They were trained in massage, hydrotherapy, electrotherapy and remedial exercises (Fletcher Little 1904).

In 1901 he established the London Institute of Massage by the Blind.

The main aims of the institute were to acquire premises staffed by visually impaired masseuses and masseurs and to convince the medical profession and the general public of the suitability of massage as a profession for visually impaired people. Fletcher Little states:

> *The Institute of Massage by the Blind has been founded with the object of organising and systematising the work of the blind operators, and rendering them entirely self-sufficient; and its root principle is to make it self-supporting by the contribution of well-paid, highly skilled operators. There is to be no flavour of charity about the work, and as soon as the institute is in full working order, it is to take its place alongside of the existing nursing institutes, agencies, etc.* (1904: 147)

In 1904 the London Institute of Massage by the Blind opened a clinic in London where many visually impaired masseuses and masseurs were employed. Initially it was dependent on public donations, but later became self-sufficient. By the time of the first annual report in 1905 the Institute had 30 qualified workers.

The London Institute of Massage by the Blind expanded and changed its name to the National Institute of Massage by the Blind in 1908; by this time there were 36 visually impaired masseuses and 21 visually impaired masseurs. In 1910 the Incorporated Society of Trained Masseuses (ISTM) (the forerunner of the Chartered Society of Physiotherapy) agreed to examine three blind men from the Hull Blind Asylum who had been trained under Dr. Fletcher Little but who wanted to acquire the Society's prestigious certificate. By this time the British and Foreign Blind Association was transcribing massage books into braille.

Dr. Fletcher Little died in 1914, and in 1915 the National Institute for Massage by the Blind, and the training of visually impaired masseuses and masseurs, was taken over by the NIB which set up its own training school, the NIB School of Massage and Electrotherapy, at Great Portland Street in London. It was designed specifically to cater for the needs of visually impaired students. In 1916 ISTM accepted for examination in massage visually impaired candidates from the NIB school, and those who succeeded received the Society's certificate in massage.

The Influence of the First and Second World Wars

The period of the First World War saw a huge expansion of the profession of massage. This expansion was not only due to appalling war injuries, including 30,000 amputations resulting from trench foot, but the poor health of young people in Britain at that time which was uncovered by the medical examinations they underwent for entry into the armed forces. Barclay states that the First World War '...would advance in an unprecedented way the cause of the Society and holistic physical therapy' (1994: 30).

The career of massage for visually impaired people was also undoubtedly boosted by the First and Second World Wars where many young men were blinded. It is stated in the Report of the Working Party on the Employment of Blind Persons:

> *In 1915 there arose the problem of the war blinded. Many of these healthy young men were eminently suitable for training as masseurs and in consultation and collaboration with St. Dunstan's the National Institute for the Blind took over the existing Institute of Massage and established its own school.* (Ministry of Labour and National Service 1951: 52)

Immediately after the First World War St. Dunstan's (a charity for war blinded servicemen and women) trained its own masseurs but the training was then taken over by the NIB. At first the NIB school catered exclusively for blinded ex-servicemen, with a few other visually impaired students being trained elsewhere, but from 1923 other visually impaired people were also trained at the school. The training lasted between 18 and two years. Tom, one of the visually impaired physiotherapists interviewed in phase one of the study remembered the differing conditions of the war blinded and civilian students after the Second World War:

> *They went under the banner of St. Dunstan's which suggested somebody who had given his sight for his country, whereas somebody like myself, who had been born partially sighted – well OK hard luck! St. Dunstan's had many millions for less than a few hundred people, whereas the NIB had thousands and thousands of people and much less money. The St. Dunstan's students had this lovely place in Park Crescent, where they were waited on by VADs, while we had a crummy hostel in New Barnet with a dreadful landlady who reported everything we did. So we were a bit antagonistic and jealous I suppose.*

Bourke (1996), in her study of the First World War, confirms that disabled ex-servicemen were given priority over disabled civilians, including children, and were given more respect. War disabled people were regarded as being the responsibility of the nation although injury was seen as more deserving than illness and white British ex-servicemen as more deserving than those of other skin colour and nationality. Their favoured position was, however, brief. Bourke states that 'By the late 1920s the respect that had initially been given to the fragmented bodies of war mutilated men had ended'(1996: 31). The quotation from Tom also suggests that people blinded in the Second World War may also have been considered more deserving that other visually impaired people at least initially. Gerber (2000), in relation to disabled veterans, comments on the constant tension between the discourses of the 'warrior' and the disabled person.

The early masseurs who were trained by St. Dunstan's worked in the military hospitals, but when these closed after the First World War St. Dunstan's helped to establish them in private practice. One venture was to open the City Clinic in London where businessmen were treated (St. Dunstan's Undated). Some of the masseurs, in order to become known and respected, were compelled initially to give their services free in their local hospitals (St. Dunstan's Review 1970).

By 1960 109 blinded ex-servicemen had been trained as physiotherapists, 37 from the First World War and 72 from the Second World War (St. Dunstan's 1960). When it is considered that 147 visually impaired people were trained as physiotherapists from 1947 to 1957 (Jenkins 1957) it becomes clear that ex-servicemen from the Second World War comprised a considerable percentage.

Most of the St. Dunstan's physiotherapists have now retired, but Howard, who was interviewed in phase one of the study, recalled the support he had been given by the organisation throughout his career:

Their help was very practical. All of my working life, until a couple of years ago, there was a sighted physio who did nothing but look after the chaps' interests – he was a bit of a dog's body you see. You could ring him up and say 'my machine's broken down' and he'd come and sort it out. He also organised our annual congress for us, and visited us every two or three months. He was someone to lean on for the practical side of things.

The Association of Blind Certified Masseurs

In 1919 the Association of Blind Certified Masseurs was formed, changing its name to the Association of Blind Chartered Physiotherapists (ABCP) in 1953, and to the Association of Visually Impaired Chartered Physiotherapists (AVICP) in 1999. Many of the original members were blinded ex-servicemen from the First World War. The aims of the Association were to provide continuing education for visually impaired masseuses and masseurs, to ensure that literature was available to them in suitable formats, and to protect their interests generally. It is stated in the 1928 annual report that the Association aims to '…promote the welfare and protect and advance the interests of qualified blind masseurs and masseuses, and to assist and secure recognition and status for them' (1928: 5).

The Association of Blind Certified Masseurs also maintained an advertising service '…so as to give wider publicity to the work, and to direct attention to the blind masseuses and masseurs in practice, not only in London, but all over the country' (Annual Report 1931: 7). Together with St. Dunstan's, they also sought work from insurance companies. Leary, a blind man who worked for many years as a lecturer at the RNIB School of Physiotherapy, sums up the work of the Association:

> *The care of the Association for its members has been demonstrated in numerous ways, such as advice and help with post-graduate services; intervention on members' behalf in instances of misunderstandings with employing authorities; advice on a vast range of personal problems; proddings in the right quarters to ensure better literature facilities; the provision of specially edited specific information; tangible help in specially needy cases; and a host of other activities. There have been numerous happy social occasions.* (1969: 6)

This association is still in existence today. Its role is both educative and social. Martin, who was interviewed in phase one of the study explained:

> *It was a means of keeping tabs on people and trying to maintain standards. It was run by the members but the RNIB had a big influence on it. It had a strong educational side to it – running courses and keeping people up to date. At first people weren't fully qualified with ultra violet, for instance, so that went through the Association.*

The membership of the association has, however, dwindled over the years and is failing to attract newly qualified physiotherapists. This can be explained in part in terms of the greater numbers of partially sighted (as opposed to blind) physiotherapists, who may need less specialised help and support. Maw (1983) notes that a high proportion of physiotherapists who attend courses run by the association are totally blind.

The termination in 1990 of the RNIB funded post of Post-Graduate Physiotherapy Officer may also have been a factor in the declining membership of the Association (French 1995). The person who occupied this part-time post kept in contact with the visually impaired physiotherapists, organised courses in co-operation with the ABCP, and offered assistance with any work-related problems the visually impaired physiotherapists encountered.

The Relationship between Visually Impaired Physiotherapists and the Chartered Society of Physiotherapy

The acceptance of visually impaired physiotherapists by the physiotherapy profession has not been easy. In 1917 two visually impaired candidates were examined in remedial exercises as well as massage by ISTM. They both passed and one of them, Mr. Percy Way, obtained the highest marks in the entire country. He became principal of the NIB School of Physiotherapy in the same year, remaining in post until 1947. So great was the opposition of ISTM to visually impaired people practising remedial exercises, however, that they declined to accept any more visually impaired candidates but instead devised a modified examination for their use (Teager 1994).

It was not just their visual impairments which created this attitude but the fact that most of them were men. The vast majority of male candidates at this time were, in fact, visually impaired although a few male nursing orderlies of the Royal Medical Corps had been permitted to take the Society's examinations since 1905. In 1916, 28 of the 31 male candidates who presented themselves for examination had visual impairments, 21 being soldiers from St. Dunstan's. Although the first men took the Society's massage examination in 1905 (Physiotherapy 1994b), male teachers were in short supply and it was still considered unseemly for women to teach men anything involving physical contact; on two occasions during 1918 members were officially reprimanded for instructing blinded soldiers (Barclay 1994). The medical profession was not in favour of masseurs either, and the rules of professional conduct, laid down in 1895 by ISTM, did not allow masseuses to massage men except in exceptional circumstances (CSP 1994b). Women instructors were, however, increasingly teaching massage and remedial exercises to servicemen, and in June 1919 the council of ISTM reluctantly agreed that this might continue (Barclay 1994).

A start was made towards the registration of men as members of ISTM in 1919 when Mr. Percy Way was co-opted to the ISTM council. Men were finally admitted as members in 1920. By 1921 there were 461 men on the Society's register out of a total membership of 7070. Although attitudes towards male masseurs gradually became more enlightened, they were only permitted to train in a limited number of physiotherapy schools (Barclay 1994). Some private schools accepted men, or catered exclusively for them, but it was not until 1932 that some hospital based schools were prepared to accept them (Thornton 1994). Even as late as 1978 only two of the nine London schools accepted men. By 1988 men still comprised only five per cent of the total membership of the CSP (Gray 1988). By 1996 the number of men had risen to approximately 11 per cent (CSP 1996).

After the Second World War the armed forces set up their own physiotherapy schools and a small splinter group of male physiotherapists broke away from the female dominated profession and set up their own association, the Society of Remedial Gymnasts, which later accepted women (Mercer 1978). Their work did not differ a great deal from that of physiotherapists, however, and in the late 1980s the two professions merged.

As the profession developed and the syllabus underwent revisions, visually impaired people were faced with more and more challenges and many adaptations to machinery were devised to allow them to continue in their practice. It was accepted that visually impaired people could master the skills of massage, but electrotherapy was barred to them until the machinery could be adapted. Several adaptations were devised including a braille galvanometer, invented by Sir Ian Fraser, which made treatments by galvanism and faradism possible, and an audible device to tune short-wave diathermy machines.

In 1946 the NIB school adopted the new curriculum of the CSP, excluding treatment with ultra-violet light (UVL) and group exercises (RNIB Undated). The training, which took three years, united the various elements of physiotherapy (massage, remedial exercises, and electrotherapy) into one course. These subjects had, until then, been taught and examined individually with separate certificates being issued for each.

Treatment with UVL was made possible by the development of the erythemameter devised by a team, led by Dr. Clive Shields, in the early 1950s. This device indicates the redness of the skin by means of audible signals. Jenkins, who was Principal of the school at the time, states:

> *In June 1954, a group of blind students gave a demonstration, using the erythemameter, to a panel of experts appointed by the Chartered Society of Physiotherapy. The results obtained by the instrument were found to be parallel with visual impression. In 1955 a further demonstration was given; this time with the technique of application of general ultra-violet irradiation. The standard of work was considered very satisfactory.* (1957: 79)

In 1956 the first visually impaired physiotherapy students were examined in the application of general UVL.

From 1956 visually impaired students followed the same curriculum as their sighted peers with the exception of focal UVL applications (for the treatment of wounds) and the supervision of large exercise groups. Until 1975 the certificate visually impaired physiotherapists received on qualification stated that the candidate had satisfied the examiners 'in accordance with the syllabus for blind candidates' but after extensive discussion between the RNIB and the CSP this clause was dropped (CSP 1975).

From the late 1970s physiotherapy courses have gradually moved to the university sector with each course being slightly different, though a core curriculum is laid down by the CSP and courses are validated by the CSP and the State Registration Board. All physiotherapists now receive a B.Sc Honours degree.

The Recognition of Visually Impaired Physiotherapists

In 1932 the NIB set up a clinic at the NIB School where electrical treatments were given; it was used by patients who found private treatment too expensive. It gave visually impaired people an opportunity to gain clinical experience and to demonstrate their competence to the public. In the 1936 annual report of the Association of Blind Certified Masseurs it states that over the course of the year there had been 5,000 attendances at the clinic. The clinic was closed in 1953 following the introduction of the NHS in 1948 which resulted in a dwindling of clients (RNIB Undated).

In 1934 the Alfred Eichholz Clinic was opened at the NIB School of Physiotherapy by means of a private donation. Its purpose was to provide visually impaired people with clinical experience and a chance to demonstrate their competence to the medical profession and the public. It is stated in the 1934 annual report of the Association of Blind Certified Masseurs that 'The chief object of the clinic is to bring before the public the special capacity of the blind for giving physical treatment, and to provide the medical profession with a convenient means of contact with blind masseurs' (1934: 7). Massage, remedial exercises, electrical treatments and bath treatments were all provided. The project was financed by William Eichholz in memory of his cousin, Alfred, who had worked extensively with blind people. It ran at a considerable loss and finally closed in 1970.

The National Health Service

Before the Second World War very few hospitals were prepared to employ visually impaired physiotherapists, although visually impaired students did receive some of their clinical education in a number of London hospitals. In 1952 a long and fruitful association began with The Whittington Hospital in Highgate which continued throughout the life of the RNIB school and NLSP (RNIB Undated). Prior to the establishment of the NHS, the NIB helped to establish visually impaired physiotherapists in private practice, usually in their own homes, by giving practical and financial assistance. Following the establishment of the NHS, however, most visually impaired physiotherapists worked in hospitals, gradually becoming accepted and independent of the NIB. By 1956 more visually impaired physiotherapists were working in hospitals than in private practice (Jenkins 1957).

The establishment of the NHS did, however, present something of a crisis for visually impaired physiotherapists, and their acceptance was hard won. In 1948 a working party was set up by the Ministry of Labour challenging the role of the visually impaired physiotherapist in an expanding profession. Points of concern were, however, overturned. It is stated in the report of the working party:

All the witnesses we have heard on the employment of blind persons as physiotherapists have agreed that there is in physiotherapy a field of useful work for blind persons. There was, however, a divergence of opinion on the extent of this field. We have found...that those without personal experience of blind workers have doubts whereas those witnesses who have worked with blind physiotherapists...have testified to their high qualities and professional competence.

> Furthermore we have received no evidence of any blind physiotherapist giving unsatisfactory service or of any difficulty being met in placing the newly-qualified in suitable appointments.

They go on to say:

> There should be no difficulty in our opinion in the profession absorbing the comparatively small number of blind persons likely to qualify...Even if ultra violet ray treatment and large group exercises are excluded from the blind physiotherapist's field, and even if other treatments requiring full vision come into use, the range still open to the blind, as experts in certain specialist treatments and otherwise, is so wide that there should continue, in the foreseeable future, to be room for as many of them as can comply with the strict requirements which those who have been responsible for their selection and training have always insisted on. (Report of the Working Party on the Employment of Blind Persons 1951: 52–53)

The Principal of the RNIB School in the 1950s, who was interviewed in phase one of the study, however, recalled considerable apprehension by managers concerning the employment of visually impaired people in hospitals:

> I had to do a lot of reassuring that the chap wasn't going to fall over as soon as he got into the department, and that he wouldn't be a liability and knock everything off the trolleys – all those sort of daft things.

Some of the physiotherapists interviewed in phase one of the study looked back to experiences of prejudice in the early years of their careers although, almost without exception, the stories they related demonstrated positive attitudes and behaviour too:

> My first superintendent was wonderful, she employed quite a few blind physiotherapists, but I had an awful job applying for jobs after that. When I went to N... the superintendent said she's got me along just to say that she'd never appoint a blind person. I said that that hardly seemed fair, and she said 'Well life's like that – don't you find that life isn't very fair?' She said I wouldn't be able to do clinics with the doctor – I'd been doing them for the past year but she wouldn't accept that. Anyway I went to B... instead where I met my husband, so there you are...but it was very frustrating at the time. (Julia)

> ...the first boss I had wouldn't promote blind people, he was quite open about it. I told the plastic surgeon who was livid, he wanted me to take up a case against the superintendent. We wrote to K... but he said it would be silly to create an atmosphere, so I backed off. The plastic surgeon was really disappointed. But I managed to get a senior job in another hospital quite easily. (Sarah)

In my first job, when I'd only been qualified a month, I was working on an orthopaedic ward and the superintendent physiotherapist told me that one of the consultants didn't want me to work on his ward. It wasn't to do with any kind of bad practice he just didn't want me there as a blind person. Anyway, the superintendent said to him 'Too bad, she's the person I've put on that ward and she's staying there' or words to that effect. The other two consultants were fine but he never was. I found it a huge thing at the time because I felt really crushed, I hadn't even done anything to give him cause for concern. (Sheila)

Thomas confirms that the acceptance of visually impaired people into the profession of physiotherapy was not easy. He states, 'Today the blind physiotherapist is recognised as a valuable member of an honourable profession, but such recognition was only won by hard work over many years' (1957: 97).

State Registration

In 1960 the Professions Supplementary to Medicine Act was passed. All physiotherapists holding qualifications from the CSP were admitted to a State Register and were entitled to refer to themselves as State Registered Physiotherapists. From 1962 State registration became a requirement of working within the NHS.

In May 1971 a working party was set up by the Council for Professions Supplementary to Medicine (CPSM) who administer the Act to investigate the situation of visually impaired people working as physiotherapists (CSP 1971a). It followed a somewhat damning inspection of the RNIB School of Physiotherapy by the CSP in January 1971 where it is stated:

A high proportion of the students appear to be studying physiotherapy from Hobson's choice rather than a burning desire to do so. A number of the students commented that they wanted a job working with people and that this seemed to be the only one available. The normal interest of physiotherapy students in the broader medical field was not apparent...The visitors feel most strongly that the whole question of training blind persons as physiotherapists should be reconsidered. (CSP 1971b)

Points of concern were, however, answered and visually impaired people continued to train and practise on the same basis as their sighted peers. Plans were, however, immediately instigated for the construction of a purpose built school for visually impaired students to offset the major criticism of the inspectors which concerned the poor premises and facilities offered at the Great Portland Street site. The new school was opened in 1978 in the grounds of the Whittington Hospital in Highgate. Teager, who became Principal of the school following the 1971 inspection, and remained in post until its closure in 1995, states 'The general acceptance of the blind physiotherapist has been hard won, is difficult to preserve, and will be constantly subject to the closest scrutiny' (1987: 135).

Beginning in 1976, physiotherapy finally became an all degree profession in 1992. In 1989, in line with other schools of physiotherapy in Britain, the North London School of Physiotherapy for the Visually Handicapped (NLSP) became affiliated to a university, the City University in London. However, despite these developments, the college enrolled its final cohort of students in 1991 and closed in 1995. The closure was due to a variety of factors including falling student numbers from both home and overseas, a greater emphasis on integration and equal opportunities within higher education, and possibly a lack of promotion and marketing (Harris 1991a).

The Demise of The North London School of Physiotherapy (NLSP)

The closure of NLSP caused much discussion and considerable alarm especially concerning the future of totally blind people wishing to enter the physiotherapy profession. Harris (1991b) reports that in a survey of physiotherapy educators not one would commit him or herself to recruiting totally blind students. A resource centre for visually impaired people wishing to become physiotherapists was, however, established in 1992 at the East London University which already had a large intake of sighted physiotherapy students. It receives extensive practical and financial backing from the RNIB and provides equipment and general support for students and university staff. This service also supports visually impaired students who wish to train as physiotherapists in other universities and employs a Physiotherapy Support Service Manager to liaise and advise students and university staff (Owen Hutchinson 1994a). In 1997 a registered blind physiotherapy student at the East London University received a first class honours degree and a prize for the best all-round student in her year (Physiotherapy Frontline 1997a).

In 1994, 24 visually impaired physiotherapy students were registered on B.Sc. degree programmes; 13 at NLSP/The City University and 11 at other universities (Owen Hutchinson 1994b). In 1998 (after the closure of NLSP) 16 visually impaired physiotherapists were enrolled in mainstream physiotherapy courses, including four totally blind students.

Visually impaired candidates for physiotherapy education are now in competition with sighted candidates for places on courses which are very popular and heavily over-subscribed. Jane Owen Hutchinson (Physiotherapy Support Service Manager), who was interviewed for this research, is of the opinion that many visually impaired people who have become physiotherapists would no longer be able to compete and that a different type of candidate, one who is more academic, is now applying than used to apply for the segregated provision. Sighted candidates may also have different characteristics from those in the past as competition has increased for them as well.

Conclusion

The college for visually impaired physiotherapy students was the only example in Britain of an institute of higher education catering specifically for disabled people. It was also the only school of physiotherapy in the world to offer a comprehensive training for visually impaired people leading to a qualification of parity with their sighted peers (RNIB 1978). This attracted many overseas students to the school providing '…a culture mix within the student body which was unique to this school, and which enriched the lives of all who taught and studied there' (Owen Hutchinson 1994a: 10). With one or two minor exceptions visually impaired students have followed the same syllabus as sighted students, and have been required to possess the same minimum entry qualifications, including (from 1983) two 'A' level GCEs.

Over the course of this century physiotherapy has become more sophisticated, technical, bureaucratic, and diverse. Physiotherapists now use a great deal of electrical equipment, they work in intensive care units, and with people who have had major surgery, serious accidents, and severe neurological damage or disease. In addition they need to cope with an increasing amount of administration and to navigate busy wards where the environment constantly changes. The fact that visually impaired people are an integral part of the physiotherapy profession can, perhaps, be viewed as an historical accident inasmuch as the profession has its roots in the tactile skill of massage which blind people traditionally practised.

The following chapter will provide a comparison between visually impaired physiotherapists and other physiotherapists using questionnaire data collected in the first phase of this study. It will include demographic details, work speciality and setting, attitudes and job satisfaction. This will provide a context for subsequent chapters which will explore the working lives of visually impaired physiotherapists and which will build upon various issues highlighted in this chapter, for example the closure of NLSP, the difficulty of using standard equipment, and the attitudes of the physiotherapy profession towards visually impaired physiotherapists.

Chapter 5

A Comparison of Visually Impaired and Sighted Physiotherapists

This chapter is based upon interview data from 45 visually impaired physiotherapists, and questionnaire data from 124 visually impaired and 198 sighted physiotherapists. It was collected during the first phase of the study. The chapter aims to provide a comparison between visually impaired and sighted physiotherapists at the end of the 1980s in terms of demographic details, aspects of employment (including speciality, grade, work setting and job satisfaction) and attitudes towards various issues including integrated physiotherapy education.

The data shows major differences between the two samples (other than that of visual impairment) and between visually impaired physiotherapists and the overall population of visually impaired people. This broad information, as well as being of interest in itself, will be of assistance when analysing the interview data which was collected in the second phase of the study. A great deal happened between phase one and phase two of the study which is likely to impinge on the working lives of visually impaired physiotherapists. In terms of legislation, the NHS and Community Care Act (1990) and the Disability Discrimination Act (1995) were both introduced and equal opportunity policies have became more widespread. Another change was that NLSP was closed in 1995 and the education of visually impaired physiotherapy students was moved to mainstream universities.

Details of Impairment

Degree of Sight

Table 5.1 shows the level of sight among the visually impaired sample as defined by the research respondents themselves. (The figures from this data have all been rounded to 0.5 or the nearest whole number.)

There is a very high proportion of totally blind people in this sample compared with the overall population of visually impaired people in Britain. Bruce et al (1991) estimate that only four per cent of registered blind people have no sight at all although this rises to 15 per cent for people aged 16 to

Table 5.1 Degree of sight of the visually impaired physiotherapists

Totally blind	41	(33%)
Light perception	9	(7%)
Minimal sight	21	(17%)
Partially sighted	51	(41%)
Other	2	(2%)

59 years (broadly those of working age). Eighteen per cent of all registered blind people have no more sight than light perception although this figure rises to 25 per cent for those aged between 16 and 59. It is perhaps the case that people with severe visual impairments are more likely to be directed towards physiotherapy, than those with more sight, as it is a well established occupation for visually impaired people (see chapter 4).

Age of Onset of Visual Impairment

Visual impairment among adults in Britain is enormously skewed to those in older age groups; it is, in fact, more age related than any other impairment, and becomes more marked the older the age group (Bruce et al 1991, Lovelock et al 1995). Ten per cent of the visually impaired population are between the ages of 16 and 59 years and 66 per cent are over the age of 75. Of those visually impaired people in the general population between the ages of 16 and 59, 30 per cent have been visually impaired from birth (Bruce et al 1991). In contrast 52 (41 per cent) of the visually impaired physiotherapists were visually impaired from birth and 112 (98 per cent) were visually impaired before the age of 25.

People who have a severe visual impairment from birth, or acquire a severe visual impairment when young, are more likely to be educated as physiotherapists than those in older age groups. The oldest person in the sample started his physiotherapy education at the age of 43. It may also be the case that visually impaired people are directed towards physiotherapy from their special schools particularly as the two grammar schools for blind children (which amalgamated in the 1980s) were administered by the RNIB as was the physiotherapy college.

Additional Impairments

Only one person in the visually impaired sample had been accepted for physiotherapy education with an additional impairment. This is in contrast to the general population of visually impaired people where a third of those between the ages of 16 and 59 have an additional impairment (Bruce et al 1991).

The lack of candidates with additional impairments is likely to have occurred because of the selection criteria of the RNIB School of Physiotherapy and NLSP. In the promotional literature of NLSP it states 'Candidates must have a record of good health and be of good physique. No candidate will be accepted for training if they have a second disability' (1981: 7). The CSP also had a policy, until the 1980s, of not admitting students with impairments on to physiotherapy courses (see chapter 3) although this was not always adhered to by individual colleges.

Demographic Details

Gender

The gender of the visually impaired and the sighted physiotherapists is shown in Table 5.2.

Table 5.2   Gender of the sighted and visually impaired physiotherapists

	Male	*Female*
Sighted physiotherapists	16 (8%)	182 (92%)
Visually impaired physiotherapists	72 (58%)	50 (40%)
No response	2 (1.5%)	– –

This table shows that whereas the proportion of sighted male physiotherapists was small, the number of visually impaired male physiotherapists exceeded visually impaired female physiotherapists. In 1996 the number of male physiotherapists in Britain was approximately 11 per cent of the total (CSP 1996). The large number of male visually impaired physiotherapists may reflect the fact that few professions have been open to visually impaired people. In addition physiotherapy was traditionally a profession offered to blinded ex-service men (see chapter 4) although most had retired by the time this study was undertaken.

Age

The sample of sighted physiotherapists was considerably younger than the sample of visually impaired physiotherapists. Three times as many visually impaired physiotherapists were over 50 years of age and nearly three times as many sighted physiotherapists were under the age of 31. This is illustrated in Table 5.3.

Table 5.3 Age of the sighted and visually impaired physiotherapists

	Under 31	Over 50
Sighted physiotherapists	74 (37%)	25 (13%)
Visually impaired physiotherapists	16 (13%)	50 (40%)

The major interpretation of this finding is that the sighted sample consisted mainly of women whereas the visually impaired sample had more men than women. Female physiotherapists are likely to leave the profession to raise children and undertake family responsibilities. The high number of visually impaired men within a profession which is predominantly female also indicates the lack of employment opportunities for visually impaired people. French (1994a) found that lack of employment opportunities was a major factor in choosing to enter the physiotherapy profession for many visually impaired men and women. It is probably also the case that visually impaired physiotherapists are less able to change their profession than sighted physiotherapists should they wish to do so.

Socio-Economic Status

Parental Occupation

The sighted and the visually impaired physiotherapists were asked to give the occupation of their father and their mother as an indication of socio-economic status. The occupations were classified into one of four categories for fathers and one of five categories for mothers as indicated in Tables 5.4 and 5.5.

It is clear, particularly from the fathers' occupations, that the sighted physiotherapists were more likely to come from professional backgrounds than the visually impaired physiotherapists. This may have reflected the greater competition experienced by sighted physiotherapists when attempting to secure a place in physiotherapy education. People from professional backgrounds have, however, always had an advantage when applying for courses in higher education and tend to acquire higher examination passes than people of lower socio-economic status (Weiner 1998).

The number of suitably qualified, visually impaired people has always been small so competition to gain a training place in their own special college, which accepted candidates until 1991, was unlikely to have been so great. This gave visually impaired physiotherapists from non-professional homes a peculiar advantage over sighted people in the same situation. Mercer (1978), in his study of the professionalisation of physiotherapists, found that 78 (41%) of his 190 research respondents came from social class

Table 5.4 Fathers' occupation of the sighted and visually impaired physiotherapists

	Sighted physiotherapists	Visually impaired physiotherapists
Professional	88 (44%)	26 (21%)
Clerical	18 (9%)	13 (10.5%)
Skilled manual	73 (37%)	64 (52%)
Unskilled manual	4 (2%)	5 (4%)
Don't know	7 (3.5%)	5 (4%)
No response	8 (4%)	11 (9%)

1 and that 24 (13 %) were related by parent or marriage to somebody already in a health care profession.

Table 5.5 Mothers' occupation of the sighted and visually impaired physiotherapists

	Sighted physiotherapists	Visually impaired physiotherapists
Professional	36 (18%)	16 (13%)
Clerical	41 (21%)	21 (17%)
Skilled manual	17 (8.5%)	20 (16%)
Unskilled manual	4 (2%)	4 (3%)
Housewife	82 (41%)	53 (43%)
Don't know	4 (2%)	3 (2%)
No response	14 (7%)	7 (6%)

Schooling

Another indication of socio-economic status relates to the types of schools the physiotherapists attended as children. Table 5.6 shows that the sighted physiotherapists were more likely to have attended private schools for at least some of their childhood. (Some people attended more than one type of school so the figures in Table 5.6 do not add up to 100 per cent.)

It is clear that the sighted physiotherapists were more likely to have attended private schools. Thirty seven per cent had attended private school for six or more years compared with 14.5 per cent of the visually impaired physiotherapists. This is complicated, however, by the fact that no private schools specifically for visually impaired children exist and it is likely that there was an unwillingness to accept visually impaired children in mainstream private schools. Mercer (1978) found that his sample of physiotherapists was overwhelmingly recruited from private schools or grammar

Table 5.6 **Types of schools attended by the sighted and visually impaired physiotherapists**

Schools	Sighted physiotherapists		Visually impaired physiotherapists	
Blind	0	(0%)	56	(45%)
Partially sighted	0	(0%)	24	(19%)
State (mainstream)	164	(83%)	76	(61%)
Private (mainstream)	74	(37%)	18	(14.5%)

schools with only six of 190 attending comprehensive schools. There has, however, been a trend away from private education for physiotherapy students today.

Physiotherapy Education

College of Physiotherapy Attended

All the visually impaired physiotherapists were educated at the RNIB School of Physiotherapy and NLSP. Two physiotherapists had started their physiotherapy education in mainstream colleges but had transferred because of lack of adequate support. The sighted sample was educated in a wide variety of colleges throughout Britain.

The existence of the 'special' college made it difficult for visually impaired candidates to be accepted elsewhere. In the CSP career literature of 1984 it is explicitly stated that 'Students with sight defects can be considered for training at the North London School of Physiotherapy for the Visually Handicapped' (1984: 2) implying that they are unlikely to be accepted elsewhere. Terry, one of the visually impaired physiotherapists interviewed in phase one of the study said:

> *I applied at two colleges. One didn't answer my letter and the other said 'You've got to go to the RNIB School' without even seeing me. It was an automatic thing 'blind and partially sighted people – that's where they go'. It's easier to send us off there than to sit down and think about what we need. I went through secondary education in an ordinary school, and did better than average, so I couldn't see why I wouldn't be able to cope in an ordinary university.*

Views of the Sighted and Visually Impaired Physiotherapists on Integrated Pre-registration Physiotherapy Education

Table 5.7 The views of the sighted and visually impaired physiotherapists on integrated pre-registration education for visually impaired physiotherapy students

The training of visually handicapped physiotherapists should remain segregated.

	Sighted physiotherapists	Visually impaired physiotherapists
Strongly disagree	5 (3%)	11 (9%)
Disagree	54 (27%)	19 (15%)
Don't know	81 (41%)	22 (18%)
Agree	46 (23%)	42 (34%)
Strongly agree	8 (4%)	30 (24%)
No response	4 (2%)	– –

The sighted and the visually impaired physiotherapists were asked for their views on integrated pre-registration education.

It is interesting that considerably more sighted physiotherapists disagreed with the segregation of physiotherapy education than visually impaired physiotherapists themselves. This may, in part, reflect the greater age of the visually impaired sample as the younger visually impaired physiotherapists were more in favour of integration than their older counterparts. Greater numbers of visually impaired physiotherapists were, however, sceptical of the process of integration, when compared with sighted physiotherapists, and were worried about the provision of braille, adapted teaching methods and other practical issues.

The visually impaired and the sighted physiotherapists who agreed with segregated provision in physiotherapy education, did so largely on the grounds of special provision and the practicalities of providing it. Below are some typical responses from a questionnaire item which asked research respondents to explain their views.

Visually Impaired Physiotherapists

> *I believe that all education of visually handicapped people is very specialised and is best undertaken in establishments where it is the norm to be blind and where special apparatus and expertise are available.*

> *Totally blind physios would be at a great disadvantage in larger mixed groups where braille, for example, may well be replaced significantly by tape. I prefer to read rather than be read to.*

Sighted Physiotherapists

> *Obviously visually handicapped physios have special educational needs and will need special equipment, for example in reading braille, and I feel it would be too expensive to incorporate this equipment into every training school.*

> *I would assume that their special needs can be best catered for in an adapted environment with teachers who are used to dealing with the blind. Providing these facilities in each physio school would be very costly and less effective.*

The visually impaired and sighted physiotherapists who disagreed with segregated provision, did so largely on the grounds of the mutual understanding and the reduction of prejudice an integrated setting may provide. Many physiotherapists from both samples also found it illogical to be educated separately when they would eventually work together. Below are some typical responses.

Visually Impaired Physiotherapists

> *Integration is the key to education and while the training remains segregated this maintains the gap between sighted and non-sighted physios. They work together in the end so why not train together?*

> *Why should the visually handicapped be segregated in training when they have to work together with the non-visually handicapped in society? Otherwise a lot of people become wary of our capabilities if we train in a protected environment.*

Sighted Physiotherapists

> *Visually handicapped still tend to be segregated by their disability. Why make this handicap more isolating when fully sighted students could also learn from them? We do in our in-service training sessions. Is this not supposed to be a caring profession?*

> *I abhor segregation of any sort. I think there may be a need for specific instruction in some areas but that is all.*

Post-registration Education

Table 5.8   Attendance at post-registration courses by the sighted and visually impaired physiotherapists

Attendance	Sighted physiotherapists	Visually impaired physiotherapists
Yes	182 (92%)	105 (84.5%)
No	14 (7%)	17 (14%)
No response	2 (1%)	2 (1.5%)

Fewer visually impaired physiotherapists attend post-registration physiotherapy courses than sighted physiotherapists. These courses may be short or long and may cover any aspect of physiotherapy. The attendance of the physiotherapists is illustrated in Table 5.8.

Some courses are run and designed specifically for visually impaired physiotherapists. The visually impaired physiotherapists were asked what sort of courses they attended. This is shown in Table 5.9.

Table 5.9   Types of courses attended by the visually impaired physiotherapists

Special courses designed for visually impaired physiotherapists	18 (14.5%)
Mainstream courses	60 (48%)
Both types of courses	53 (43%)

Because of the small number of visually impaired physiotherapists, courses run specifically for them offer less variety of subject matter than general courses which are open to all physiotherapists. Course programmes for visually impaired physiotherapists have, over the years, been orientated to out-patient work.

The visually impaired physiotherapists were asked whether any special needs they had were met on general post-registration courses and those run specifically for them. This is illustrated in Table 5.10.

It can be seen that 41 per cent of visually impaired physiotherapists who attended general courses believed that their needs were never or only occasionally met compared with 16.5 per cent who attended courses designed specifically for visually impaired physiotherapists. The major issue revealed by the sample was lack of an alternative to visual displays such as the blackboard, overhead projector and slides. Lack of time, problems of orientation in a strange environment and lack of braille and large print materials were also noted. These findings were very similar to those reported by Simkiss et al (1998) and reflect the types of barriers

Table 5.10 The degree to which the needs of the visually impaired physiotherapists were met on post-registration courses

If you attend courses run specifically for visually handicapped physiotherapists, or primarily for sighted physiotherapists, do you find that any special needs you have are adequately catered for?

	General courses		Specific courses	
Never	10	(10%)	1	(1.5%)
Occasionally	41	(39%)	9	(15%)
I have no special needs	12	(12%)	8	(13%)
Usually	36	(35%)	31	(51%)
Always	3	(3%)	12	(20%)

highlighted in the social model of disability. The following quotations illustrate some typical responses from a questionnaire item which asked research respondents to explain their views.

Excessive reliance on slides or blackboard with no certainty of being able to sit in a position to see or adequate explanation when I can't.

Course material are not available in braille or on tape.

Blind people can't keep up with sighted people.

Employment

Work Setting

Table 5.11 indicates the work settings of the sighted and the visually impaired physiotherapists. Some of the physiotherapists worked in more than one setting.

This analysis shows that a similar number of visually impaired and sighted physiotherapists worked in hospitals but far more visually impaired physiotherapists worked in private practice particularly on a full-time basis (many physiotherapists combine private practice with hospital work). Totally blind men, in particular, were more likely than other physiotherapists to run full-time private practices. The interview data in phase one of the study showed that blind male physiotherapists worked in private practice both for financial reasons and to create a more controlled and affable environment. This is illustrated in the following quotations from interviews undertaken with private practitioners:

Table 5.11 The work settings of the sighted and visually impaired physiotherapists

	Sighted physiotherapists		Visually impaired physiotherapists	
Hospital	137	(70%)	83	(67%)
Private practice	33	(17%)	51	(41%)
Community	49	(20%)	9	(7%)
Health centre	14	(7%)	2	(2%)
College (teaching)	6	(3%)	8	(6%)

I always had private work as my aim because its a lot more efficient working from your own home rather than a busy hospital department...you can be extremely efficient in a small area but in a hospital ward with trolleys around, drugs on it, that sort of thing, I don't think it's suitable for people who are blind. (Henry)

My motivation was to earn more money. I have a wife and three daughters and my salary wasn't enough to have a mortgage and so on. Two months later I was more than doubling my previous salary. I'll own up, I love having money. So money was my motive, but I had to work very hard. (Tom)

It was noted by Bruce et al (1991) and Sly (1996) in chapter 2 that a higher proportion of disabled people, than non-disabled people, are self-employed.

About three times as many sighted physiotherapists worked in the community. The lower numbers of visually impaired people in community work probably reflects difficulties of transportation and changing environments; many advertisements for community posts insist that applicants can drive. More visually impaired physiotherapists worked as lecturers than sighted physiotherapists although the numbers are very small in both groups. The larger numbers in the visually impaired sample may have been due to the age and gender differences between the two samples.

Work Specialities

One hundred and forty seven (74%) of the sighted physiotherapists and 88 (71%) of the visually impaired physiotherapists had specialised in particular areas of physiotherapy. Those who had specialised were asked to identify their area or areas of specialisation. Up to four specialities per person were coded. This is illustrated in Table 5.12.

Visually impaired physiotherapists were far more likely to specialise in general out-patient work, including sports medicine and manipulations, than sighted physiotherapists. This type of work provides a physically more controlled environment, compared with ward or community work, and is

Table 5.12 The work specialities of the sighted and visually impaired physiotherapists

	Sighted physiotherapists		Visually impaired physiotherapists	
General out-patients	60	(30%)	76	(61%)
Sports injuries	14	(7%)	29	(23%)
Neurology	32	(16%)	10	(7%)
Manipulations	20	(10%)	52	(42%)
Paediatrics	41	(21%)	6	(5%)
Obstetrics and gynaecology	25	(13%)	6	(5%)
Teaching	6	(3%)	8	(6%)
Management	16	(8%)	17	(14%)

the type of work undertaken in private practice. These differences, particularly with regard to private practice, may also have reflected the large number of men in the visually impaired sample and the fact that the visually impaired sample was older than the sighted sample – they would have had more time and experience to set up private practices.

The higher numbers of visually impaired physiotherapists in teaching and management may have reflected the differences in the samples with regard to gender and age. The lack of visually impaired physiotherapists who worked in the area of obstetrics and gynaecology is likely to have reflected the high number of men in the visually impaired sample as this is work usually undertaken by female physiotherapists.

There has been some resistance to accepting visually impaired physiotherapists on post-registration courses, particularly those concerning neurology and paediatrics, which may have accounted in part for the lower numbers of visually impaired physiotherapists who had specialised in these fields (French 1990a, 1995). As will be seen later, however, visually impaired people do consider paediatrics to be a particularly difficult field, although some people have worked successfully in this area.

Full-time and Part-time Work

Table 5.13 shows the numbers of sighted and visually impaired physiotherapists in full-time and part-time work.

The greater number of visually impaired physiotherapists who worked full-time probably reflects the gender and age difference in the samples as young women are more likely to leave the profession to raise children. There were far more young women in the sighted sample.

Table 5.13 Full-time and part-time work of the sighted and visually impaired physiotherapists

	Sighted physiotherapists	Visually impaired physiotherapists
Full-time	114 (57.5%)	96 (77%)
Part-time	70 (35%)	27 (22%)
No response	14 (7%)	1 (1%)

Job Satisfaction

The questionnaire contained 22 items on different aspects of job satisfaction. Both samples showed a high level of satisfaction with little difference between them. This is shown in Tables 5.14 and 5.15.

The job satisfaction data further illustrated that the visually impaired sample were more satisfied than the sighted sample with their pre-registration education, their salary, their promotion prospects and their working conditions (French 1994a). This may have reflected the fact that a higher percentage were working in private practice. They may also have been comparing themselves with other disabled or visually impaired people; that is, their expectations of employment may have been lower than that of the sighted sample (French 1994a).

With some other questionnaire items regarding job satisfaction, however, visually impaired physiotherapists were more likely to be 'satisfied' than 'very satisfied' when compared with the sighted physiotherapists. These areas of job satisfaction included, the nature of the work, interest in the work, sense of achievement, level of responsibility, variety, enjoyment of work and colleagues, and contact with patients.

Table 5.14 Job satisfaction of the sighted and visually impaired physiotherapists

Taking your job as a whole what best describes your feelings about it?

	Sighted physiotherapists	Visually impaired physiotherapists
1 Like it very much	92 (46%)	52 (42%)
2	82 (41%)	54 (43.5%)
3	22 (11%)	16 (13%)
4	1 (0.5%)	1 (1%)
5 Hate it	1 (0.5%)	1 (1%)

Table 5.15 Job satisfaction of the sighted and visually impaired physiotherapists

How satisfied are you with your present job?

	Sighted physiotherapists	Visually impaired physiotherapists
Very satisfied	64 (32%)	44 (35%)
Satisfied	85 (43%)	52 (42%)
Neutral	29 (15%)	15 (12%)
Dissatisfied	12 (6%)	6 (5%)
Very dissatisfied	4 (2%)	4 (3%)
No response	4 (2%)	3 (2%)

Whereas 13 (6.5%) of the sighted physiotherapists admitted to wanting to change their profession, 19 (15%) of the visually impaired physiotherapists wanted to do so. And whereas 30 (15%) of the sighted physiotherapists had doubts about the value of physiotherapy, 29 (23%) of the visually impaired physiotherapists had such doubts. Twenty one (17%) of the visually impaired physiotherapists, compared with 11 (5.5%) of the sighted physiotherapists, felt under-stimulated intellectually at work. It is possible that age and gender were having an effect on the way people felt about their work. The fact that visually impaired people have less choice of occupation than non-disabled people may also have accounted for this effect (French 1994a). Despite the general high level of satisfaction among the visually impaired physiotherapists, most claimed that they would not have become physiotherapists if they were sighted. This is illustrated in Table 5.16.

It can be seen that 66 per cent of the visually impaired physiotherapists did not think they would choose to be physiotherapists if they were fully sighted. Nevertheless, most of the visually impaired sample believed that physiotherapy was the best choice for them. This is illustrated in Table 5.17.

Table 5.16 Choice of physiotherapy as a career for the visually impaired physiotherapists

Do you think you would be a physiotherapist if you could see normally?

Definitely not	43 (35%)
Probably not	38 (31%)
Don't know	11 (9%)
Probably	21 (17%)
Definitely	7 (5%)
No response	4 (3%)

Table 5.17 Satisfaction of the sighted and visually impaired physiotherapists with physiotherapy as a career

Physiotherapy was the best career choice for me.

	Sighted physiotherapists		Visually impaired physiotherapists	
Definitely not	1	(0.5%)	3	(2%)
Probably not	9	(4.5%)	7	(6%)
Don't know	13	(6.5%)	4	(3%)
Probably	88	(44%)	45	(36%)
Definitely	87	(44%)	65	(52%)

When asked to explain their views many of the visually impaired physiotherapists spoke in terms of the limited choice of work available to them. Below are some typical responses:

Given the choice of careers in 1969 normally available to a totally blind person, physiotherapy was the best.

It was the only career that would allow me to work with people in the medical field.

It was either physio or computers, and I can't stand computers.

It was the only career on offer that was not sedentary.

Some of the physiotherapists who became visually impaired in adulthood found that physiotherapy was the closest approximation they could get to their previous profession:

If my vision had not deteriorated greatly in my early twenties I would have remained in work as a teacher.

Continuation of paramedical theme, as failing eyesight meant that dentistry was no longer possible.

In view of my visual handicap at age 22, physiotherapy was an ideal second career. I was a Registered Mental Nurse.

Before being blinded I was a structural engineer. With physiotherapy the structures apply to the body.

Others felt that they would not have thought of physiotherapy as a career if it had not been for their visual impairments.

Grade

Table 5.18 Employment grades of the sighted and visually impaired physiotherapists

	Sighted physiotherapists	*Visually impaired physiotherapists*
Junior	24 (12%)	12 (10%)
Senior	120 (60%)	55 (44%)
Superintendent	25 (13%)	15 (12%)
District Manager	1 (0.5)	4 (3%)
Lecturer	2 (1%)	2 (2%)

The grades of the sighted and the visually impaired physiotherapists are shown in Table 5.18. (Some of the physiotherapists were in private practice and, therefore, had no grade.)

Slightly more visually impaired physiotherapists were in district manager and lecturing posts, which probably reflected their gender and greater age. It takes time to achieve these posts and male physiotherapists are disproportionately represented in management positions (CSP 1996).

Although the visually impaired physiotherapists do appear to compare favourably with the sighted physiotherapists with regard to grade, some visually impaired physiotherapists believed that their promotion prospects had been adversely affected by factors related to visual impairment. This is shown in Table 5.19.

Table 5.19 Promotion prospects of the visually impaired physiotherapists

My promotion prospects have been adversely affected because of my visual handicap.

Strongly agree	14 (11%)
Agree	33 (27%)
Don't know	16 (13%)
Disagree	33 (27%)
Strongly disagree	22 (18%)
No response	6 (5%)

Thirty eight per cent of visually impaired physiotherapists believed that their promotion prospects had been adversely affected by factors related to visual impairment largely because of other people's attitudes and behaviour. Below are some responses to a questionnaire item which asked them to explain:

> *I have been refused an interview because of my visual handicap. I was told the hospital I wanted to work in was unsuitable for blind people.*

> *I feel that promotion has only been gained in the absence of suitably qualified, sighted opposition.*

Similar comments were made during the interviews:

> *If there are other competitors who have full vision I think it is difficult. If people don't know and are not prepared to give you the opportunity to sell yourself it's difficult, you can't do it at an interview. (Stephen)*

> *Four interviews for high grade posts in the past five years and, I don't know, you just wonder sometimes, you're convinced that you are eligible for these positions...you begin to hear the same things too often 'It was a very close thing, you were a very good contender but...' (Malcolm)*

Seventy seven (62%) of the visually impaired physiotherapists said they had avoided promotion because of their visual impairment. Of the 17 people who provided an open response to this questionnaire item, 15 mentioned administration as being the major deterrent to promotion and two mentioned problems of speed. This is illustrated in the following responses:

> *I accepted the post of designated district physio but had to resign as I found it too difficult to keep up with the increased load of paper work.*

> *I have avoided promotion knowing full well that I would not handle the clerical and administrative work and the responsibilities required.*

The fact that visually impaired physiotherapists are able to achieve senior positions may reflect, in part, the continual shortage of physiotherapists within the NHS. As noted in chapter 2 a shortage of workers, for example at times of war, provides opportunities for disabled people to find employment.

Number of Posts in the Careers of the Physiotherapists

The physiotherapists were asked how many posts they had had in their careers. This is illustrated in Table 5.20.

Table 5.20 Number of posts in the careers of the sighted and visually impaired physiotherapists

Number of Posts	Sighted physiotherapists	Visually impaired physiotherapists
1	4 (2%)	7 (6%)
2	32 (16%)	14 (11%)
3	33 (17%)	27 (22%)
4	33 (17%)	25 (20%)
5	31 (16%)	15 (12%)
6	24 (12%)	15 (12%)
7	12 (6%)	8 (6%)
8	11 (5%)	2 (2%)
9	3 (1%)	5 (4%)
10	6 (3%)	2 (2%)
No response	10 (5%)	4 (3%)

There appears to be little difference between the samples, but considering that the visually impaired sample was older, there may have been a tendency for them to change their jobs less frequently than the sighted physiotherapists. This is likely to have reflected the greater numbers of visually impaired physiotherapists in private practice and possibly greater difficulty in securing new posts and gaining promotion. It appears, however, that despite the added difficulties visually impaired people experience in negotiating new environments, they were not deterred from changing jobs.

Attitudes towards Visually Impaired Physiotherapists

Perceptions of the Attitude of the Physiotherapy Profession towards Visually Impaired Physiotherapists

The sighted and the visually impaired physiotherapists were asked whether the physiotherapy profession welcomes visually impaired physiotherapists. This is illustrated in Table 5.21.

The sighted sample felt more positive about the attitude of the physiotherapy profession towards visually impaired physiotherapists than the visually impaired physiotherapists themselves. The discrepancy between the two samples may indicate a lack of understanding among sighted physiotherapists about the problems visually impaired physiotherapists encounter. Below are a selection of responses from the visually impaired physiotherapists who agreed or disagreed that they are welcomed by their profession.

Table 5.21 Perceptions of the attitude of the physiotherapy profession towards visually impaired physiotherapists

The physiotherapy profession welcomes visually handicapped physiotherapists.

	Sighted physiotherapists	Visually impaired physiotherapists
Strongly disagree	1 (.5%)	3 (2%)
Disagree	7 (3.5%)	42 (34%)
Don't know	77 (39%)	33 (27%)
Agree	89 (45%)	44 (35%)
Strongly agree	22 (11%)	2 (2%)
No response	2 (1%)	

Agree

> *I have always been accepted as a chartered physiotherapist who happens to be blind rather than a blind chartered physiotherapist.*

> *The profession acknowledges the contribution the visually impaired can make.*

Disagree

> *There is a lack of understanding or even the desire to understand what a visually handicapped person can do. Too many preconceived ideas. I got turned down from a job because someone decided I wouldn't manage but I couldn't defend myself.*

> *If blind physiotherapists had not become established in the period of sympathy during World War 1 I don't believe it would now exist, owing to the attitudes of sighted physios.*

The sighted physiotherapists often based their judgement on their personal experiences of working with visually impaired physiotherapists and many viewed the existence of the special training college as an indication of acceptance, rather than lack of acceptance, of visually impaired physiotherapists by the profession. Below are a selection of their responses:

Agree

> *I have worked with three blind/partially sighted physiotherapists. They have always been happy in their work, taken a full work load and been respected by their colleagues.*

They must be welcome because there is a school for blind and partially sighted students.

Disagree

I have mixed feelings on this subject. I have found the visually handicapped both accepted well and barely tolerated by different superintendents.

I have seen various reactions to visually handicapped physiotherapists by other staff – some excellent, some intolerant.

The Perceived Abilities of Blind and Visually Impaired Physiotherapists

Both samples were asked whether they thought it was possible for blind and partially sighted physiotherapists to work successfully in all areas of physiotherapy. There was considerable disagreement between the samples as shown in Tables 5.22 and 5.23.

Table 5.22   The abilities of blind physiotherapists as viewed by the sighted and visually impaired physiotherapists

It is possible for blind physiotherapists to work successfully in all specialities.

	Sighted physiotherapists	Visually impaired physiotherapists
Agree	22 (11%)	28 (22%)
Disagree	109 (55%)	71 (57%)
Don't know	66 (33%)	25 (20%)
No response	1 (0.5%)	– –

Table 5.23   The abilities of partially sighted physiotherapists as viewed by the sighted and visually impaired physiotherapists

It is possible for partially sighted physiotherapists to work successfully in all specialities.

	Sighted physiotherapists	Visually impaired physiotherapists
Agree	64 (32%)	62 (50%)
Disagree	45 (23%)	91 (15%)
Don't know	87 (44%)	39 (31%)
No response	2 (1%)	4 (3%)

The visually impaired sample were more positive about their own abilities than the sighted sample were towards them, and the sighted sample showed less certainty with more in the 'don't know' category. Both samples are more positive about the abilities of partially sighted physiotherapists to work successfully in all specialities than blind physiotherapists. The abilities of visually impaired people is frequently doubted and this increases with the severity of the impairment (Simkiss et al 1998). The uncertainty of their colleagues, concerning the ability of visually impaired physiotherapists to fulfil their role, has the potential to cause employment problems especially if the doubtful person is in a position of power.

Interesting differences and similarities emerged concerning the specialities in which the physiotherapists thought blind and partially sighted physiotherapists were unsuitable. These are shown in Tables 5.24 and 5.25.

Table 5.24   Perceptions of the sighted and visually impaired physiotherapists on the ability of blind physiotherapists to cope in various specialities

Specialities with which blind physiotherapists cannot cope.

	Sighted physiotherapists	Visually impaired physiotherapists
Paediatrics	38 (19%)	58 (47%)
Intensive care	108 (54.5%)	87 (70%)
Hydrotherapy	30 (15%)	0 (0%)
Neurology	11 (5.5%)	4 (3%)

Table 5.25   Perceptions of the sighted and visually impaired physiotherapists on the ability of partially sighted physiotherapists to cope in various specialities

Specialities with which partially sighted physiotherapists cannot cope.

	Sighted physiotherapists	Visually impaired physiotherapists
Paediatrics	24 (12%)	57 (46%)
Intensive care	99 (50%)	65 (52%)
Hydrotherapy	13 (6.5%)	0 (0%)
Neurology	26 (13%)	1 (1%)

There was considerable agreement between the two samples regarding the capability of blind and partially sighted physiotherapists to work in intensive care units; the visually impaired sample were, in fact, rather less positive. In contrast there was considerable disagreement regarding the capability of blind and partially sighted physiotherapists to work in hydrotherapy, paediatrics and neurology. Like other physiotherapists, most of the visually impaired physiotherapists were compelled to work within intensive care units during weekend and 'on-call' evening rotas during the early years of their careers. Some of the responses of the visually impaired physiotherapists are given below:

> *A busy ITU (intensive therapy unit) is not an area that I feel confident or comfortable in. Good vision seems vital to me for full-time ITU work.*
>
> *Treatment of bedsores and open wounds – impossible to successfully implement an aseptic technique for a blind physiotherapist.*
>
> *Community physiotherapy; the travelling would be difficult. So would the necessity to constantly cope with different surroundings.*
>
> *Difficult to manage children who may be active and poor communicators.*

The responses of the sighted physiotherapists indicate that they regarded a much wider range of specialities unsuitable for visually impaired physiotherapists. Some even doubted the ability of visually impaired physiotherapists to 'find their way around'. Some of the sighted physiotherapists, in addition, perceived the visually impaired physiotherapists as unsafe, both with regard to themselves and with regard to their patients and clients, in a wide range of situations. This is something the visually impaired physiotherapists rarely said about themselves. Some responses of the sighted physiotherapists are given below:

> *I don't feel that a blind person could cope with a busy ward with a high turnover – where you never find the same patient in the same place. Too much adaptation would be needed.*
>
> *It would be difficult for a blind physio to work in a high tech environment where attention to monitors and visual displays is important.*
>
> *Geriatrics where the patient may be falling or unable to communicate verbally.*
>
> *Hydrotherapy or any speciality where observation of a patient is paramount to safety.*

Unless they have a helper with them all the time, things like wet floors on wards make me nervous.

Children are unpredictable and could possibly come to harm while being treated...In emergencies a sighted person would cope more quickly.

These and other comments, taken collectively, exclude most areas of physiotherapy to visually impaired people. The presumption that disabled people are unsafe, both to themselves and others, has been highlighted by Barnes (1991) and Zarb (1995a) and is likely to be experienced as very oppressive. It must be remembered, however, that many of the physiotherapists had had little or no experience of working with a visually impaired colleague. Nevertheless, such attitudes have the potential to create considerable barriers for visually impaired physiotherapists.

The Perceived Suitability of Physiotherapy as a Career for Blind and Partially Sighted People

The physiotherapists were asked whether physiotherapy was a suitable career for blind and partially sighted people. Their responses are shown in Tables 5.26 and 5.27.

The sighted physiotherapists were less certain about the suitability of physiotherapy as a career for blind and partially sighted people though very few stated that the career was unsuitable. More sighted physiotherapists than visually impaired physiotherapists stated that they did not know. More positive attitudes were shown towards partially sighted than blind physiotherapists by both samples, and the visually impaired physiotherapists were more positive in their attitudes than the sighted physiotherapists.

Table 5.26 The perceived suitability of physiotherapy as a career for blind people

	Sighted physiotherapists	Visually impaired physiotherapists
Unsuitable	1 (0.5%)	1 (1%)
Probably unsuitable	1 (3.3%)	1 (1%)
Don't know	22 (11%)	2 (2%)
Probably suitable	99 (50%)	28 (22.5%)
Suitable	62 (31%)	90 (72.5%)
No response	3 (1.5%)	2 (2%)

90   *Disabled People and Employment*

Table 5.27   The perceived suitability of physiotherapy as a career for partially sighted people

	Sighted physiotherapists		Visually impaired physiotherapists	
Unsuitable	0	(0%)	0	(0%)
Probably unsuitable	5	(2.5%)	0	(0%)
Don't know	15	(7.5%)	6	(5%)
Probably suitable	87	(44%)	18	(4.5%)
Suitable	88	(44%)	96	(77%)
No response	3	(1.5%)	4	(3%)

The Perceived Difficulty of Physiotherapy as a Career for Blind and Partially Sighted People

The physiotherapists were asked whether physiotherapy had become more difficult for visually impaired physiotherapists over the years. Table 5.28 gives their responses.

Table 5.28   The views of the sighted and visually impaired physiotherapists on the difficulty of physiotherapy as a career for visually impaired people

Over the years do you consider that the situation for visually handicapped physiotherapists has become?

	Sighted physiotherapists		Visually impaired physiotherapists	
More difficult	41	(21%)	62	(50%)
Easier	13	(6.5%)	16	(13%)
The same	32	(16%)	18	(14.5%)
Don't know	108	(54.5%)	24	(19%)
No response	4	(2%)	4	(3%)

Half of the sample of visually impaired physiotherapists considered that their situation had become more difficult over the years compared with only 21 per cent of the sighted physiotherapists. The sighted physiotherapists may have underestimated the difficulties visually impaired people experience. Most of the barriers experienced by the visually impaired physiotherapists were environmental including inaccessible equipment, increased administration and the inability to drive a car. Below are some of their responses:

More Difficult

Electro-medical equipment is becoming increasingly 'high-tech' – i.e. with flat panel controls and we have to shop around more to find appropriate equipment.

Increase in pace of work in NHS hospitals.

Increased use of general documentation, and the introduction of more sophisticated equipment.

Physiotherapists are under greater academic pressure than pioneer blind physiotherapists.

It is more difficult because more jobs require ability to drive a car.

The minority of the visually impaired physiotherapists who thought the job had become easier spoke mainly in terms of increased acceptance and more positive attitudes.

Easier

Handicap in general is more acceptable than it has been. The government has provided help in practical terms and attitudes change with experience.

As more and more visually handicapped people qualify and work in the NHS, they become more acceptable to working colleagues.

Twenty five years ago it was much more difficult for visually impaired persons to get jobs.

We have become more widely accepted now due to many highly successful visually handicapped physios.

Conclusion

This chapter has highlighted many differences and similarities, between the two samples of physiotherapists. The variation within the samples was also marked. The visually impaired sample differed from the sighted sample in various ways other than visual impairment, for example in age, gender and social class. They also had little choice but to train in their own special college. Both samples specialised in diverse areas of physiotherapy but there were greater numbers of visually impaired physiotherapists in out-patient settings and private practice and fewer working in the community.

Although some differences were noted, the two samples were very similar in terms of grade and job satisfaction and in the number of jobs they had had. The visually impaired sample reported, however, that their promotion prospects had been adversely affected by factors related to visual impairment and that their choice of profession had been very restricted. The visually impaired physiotherapists gave many examples of the barriers they encountered at all levels of post-registration education and employment.

The sighted and visually impaired physiotherapists differed in the meaning they attached to visual impairment, although the variation within the two samples was marked. The sighted sample were more positive about integrated physiotherapy education than the visually impaired sample although they were also less sure. Some of the sighted sample felt that visually impaired physiotherapists were unsafe although visually impaired physiotherapists rarely said this about themselves. The sighted physiotherapists felt considerably more confident than the visually impaired physiotherapists that the physiotherapy profession welcomes visually impaired physiotherapists.

The visually impaired physiotherapists were clearly subject to attitudinal, environmental and structural barriers as described in chapter 1. They were working and studying in settings, and within an attitudinal climate, that was not always conducive to their needs. Despite this, their job satisfaction and position within the profession was on a par with their sighted colleagues.

The following four chapters, on post-registration education and the employment experiences of visually impaired physiotherapists, are written largely from the interview data collected in phase two of the study. These chapters will build on the data provided here by investigating in detail the barriers visually impaired physiotherapists experience at work and the ways in which they minimise, overcome or manage these barriers. These chapters will provide an opportunity to examine if and how the working lives of the visually impaired physiotherapists changed over a period of eight years, during which time the NHS and Community Care Act (1990) and the Disability Discrimination Act (1995) were passed.

Chapter 6

Educational Inclusion: Barriers and Coping Strategies

This chapter will explore the barriers to post-registration courses and mainstream education for visually impaired physiotherapists and the strategies they adopt to overcome or reduce these barriers. It is based on the 20 interviews undertaken in the second phase of the study. Post-registration education is essential to all physiotherapists who wish to advance their careers. It was noted in chapter 1 that evidence of continuing professional development will soon be required in order for physiotherapists to renew their state registration and to work within the NHS. The visually impaired physiotherapists highlighted post-registration education as a vital aspect of their working lives, in terms, for example, of promotion.

Most of the physiotherapists interviewed (16 of the 20) spoke of the barriers they face in post-registration education and the strategies they use to cope with these barriers. Disabling barriers in adult education have been highlighted by many researchers with regard to disabled people generally (for example French 1988, Myers and Parker 1996, Leicester and Lovett 1997, Ash et al 1998, Borland and James 1999) and visually impaired people specifically (for example French 1990b, Simkiss et al 1998, Owen Hutchinson et al 1998). Talking of visually impaired students Simkiss et al state:

The focus groups provide testimony that not only does the learning support available to visually impaired pupils and students demonstrate major shortcomings, including a lack of sensitivity to and accommodation of individuals' requirements, but also that specific learning strategies designed to enhance achievement appear to be absent. (1998: 87)

Individual disabled people have also given their accounts of disabling barriers in adult education. McDonald, for example, states:

I was alone as a disabled student and most of the time these establishments relied on me to educate both students and staff about disability issues and also to raise the general level of disability awareness. (1996: 126)

Similarly, a blind university student states:

> *It was a great struggle...all the time I had to fight for it, asking for book lists in advance, reading things from the board – it was constant. I had to be very assertive and they didn't like it because they thought I was being really awkward and persistent...the course was new so there was nothing in braille or on tape. I had to teach them. I had to teach the library staff how to help me.* (French et al 1997)

Myers and Parker (1996) believe that disabled students are likely to encounter physical, financial and attitudinal barriers in higher education and that a great deal of work has yet to be done if disabled students are to participate fully.

The educational programmes the physiotherapists mentioned varied, ranging from Masters Degrees and professional courses, such as courses in manipulations and sports injuries, to in-service education and occasional lectures, demonstrations and practical workshops. Many of the barriers to education reflect those which the visually impaired physiotherapists highlighted in phase one of the study (see chapter 5 and French 1990b) and indicate that little substantial change has taken place over the eight year period between phases one and two of the study.

The particular barriers the visually impaired physiotherapists encountered will now be discussed together with the strategies they used to overcome, minimise or manage them.

Barriers

Visual Teaching Aids

A major barrier highlighted by the physiotherapists was the use of visual aids, such as slides, blackboards and overhead projectors, without any alternatives. Demonstrations of practical techniques posed similar problems. Andrea explained:

> *Everything is terribly, terribly visual, it's all overhead things and slides and, you know, people seem incapable of doing a talk without visual cues all the time...They don't think about what I need. They don't acknowledge it. Well jokingly, when it's our people, they say 'Can everybody see that?' and I say 'No'. Everyone titters, but nobody ever says they're sorry or anything like that. Occasionally they ask if I would like them to read it out, they at least realise that I'm there, but that's about it really.*

Sheila related similar experiences:

> *One lecture in particular sticks in my memory where they were using an overhead projector, or it might have been slides, and the person would just refer to 'number such and such' she would make no verbal description of it at all and I was absolutely lost.*

Another barrier encountered by some of the physiotherapists was the lack of an alternative to standard print, such as large print, braille and audiotape. Josephine said:

> *I find there is nothing much in braille really. I went on a course and he handed around sheets all the time and it was useless because there was no time to get it read. I felt it was a waste of time.*

The physiotherapists who could not use print were often responsible for sorting the problem out for themselves. Sarah explained:

> *On the last course I did, on the sacro-iliac joint, I got the stuff brailled, but it came back as I don't know how many sheets, it came in a great big box and I got it months later.*

The only time the physiotherapists were provided with literature in braille was when courses were run by the ABCP. There is a vastly reduced number of books in braille, large print and on audiotape when compared with those in standard print. Robert said:

> *You're on your own aren't you? Books in the areas I'm interested in are very limited in braille, very limited. So you get what you can, and use the close-circuit TV and anyone who is willing to read.*

The inaccessibility of written materials is a common problem for visually impaired children and students (French and Swain 1997, French et al 1997). Visually impaired people need a variety of alternatives to standard print, according to their level of sight and individual preferences. These include large print, audiotape and braille. The importance of providing educational materials in a suitable format is emphasised by Curtis et al. They state:

> *It is vital that training programmes are delivered at an appropriate level with information and instruction provided in a format which visually impaired trainees can access. There can be a tendency, with visually impaired trainees, to place too much emphasis on verbal communication and it is important that they should not have to rely totally on memory and miss out on written communication.* (1997: 13–4)

They also emphasise the importance of giving teaching staff extra time to meet the needs of visually impaired students.

Speed of Teaching

Some of the physiotherapists found the pace of courses too fast and were conscious of the possibility of holding other people up. Malcolm explained:

I have to admit that one feels 'Oh dear, am I going to slow the whole thing down and get in the way?', that sort of thing, particularly these days when things seem to move so fast...they whiz on, it all flies on.

Sarah misses out on information because of the speed at which courses move and felt that this may adversely affect the way she is perceived by colleagues:

One course I went on recently, the chap went through it at such a rate of knots that I did miss out quite a bit. As a senior you are expected to do your part in the teaching and if you say, 'I don't feel happy to teach that because I didn't grasp it all' it reflects back on you. You're the one that looks inadequate. People have never understood.

Julia takes a facilitator on courses with her because she found, among other things, that her note taking in braille was too slow:

I'd never quite realised how slow I was at note taking in braille. I've always dotted quite fast but I couldn't possibly write at the same speed as the facilitator could. So she used to take all the notes down and then read it on to tape for me at night so that I could get the cassette the next day and copy it up.

The fact that visually impaired people and disabled people generally take longer to perform many tasks was highlighted in chapter 2. Talking of disabled social work students Baron et al state:

One constant theme was the need to have more time than other students to complete tasks...programmes had not grasped this nettle and developed systems of allowing different routes and time-scales leading to the same destination. The possibility of disabled students producing work of the same quality as students without such impairments was thus reduced. (1996: 372)

Not only does this extra time requirement make learning within a group difficult but, as the physiotherapists point out, it can give rise to awkward social situations which may affect how they feel about themselves and how other people view them.

Travelling to Courses and Coping with the Venue

Some of the physiotherapists, particularly those who are totally blind, found the difficulty of the journey and managing in a strange environment, inhibitory factors in attending post-registration courses. Andrea said:

> *It's the hassle of getting there and getting back again and finding your way around if you are on your own in a strange place...It's always been OK but nobody ever said they would help or meet me at the station...it's just the fear of going to these things on your own.*

John gave details of a traumatic journey he made to a hospital where a course was being held. He is critical of the lack of help he received:

> *As you get older going on courses is a problem. I went on a course a few years ago...and I specifically asked, first of all was there anybody going there who was coming from my side of town, and what about directions from the station, all that sort of thing. When I got off the train it was snowing, there wasn't a bloody soul in sight, so I didn't even know which way to go to get out of the station...I was just fuming when I thought how physiotherapists are supposed to be sympathetic because I was more or less abandoned as a totally blind person...I was late and I was flying along the road and I crashed head first into this bloody bus stop and had a lump the size of an egg on my head when I got there and I was really annoyed with them because they could, without very much effort, have been a hell of a lot more helpful.*

It might be expected that as the visually impaired physiotherapists and the sighted physiotherapists are colleagues, with equal status, that attitudes and behaviour towards the visually impaired physiotherapists would be positive (McConkey and McCormack 1983). However many of the physiotherapists spoke of insensitive attitudes and behaviour and lack of understanding.

Alice, whose sight has gradually deteriorated over the years, is very daunted by courses in terms of coping with the journey and the unfamiliar environment. Like John, she equates the problem, in part, to 'getting older':

> *I have all these inhibitions. In fact if I didn't have Sam (husband) to take me to things, or another sighted person, I just wouldn't go because I'm too blind to get around in unfamiliar settings. I can't find my way and I get very, very anxious and I hate it if I'm thrown into a completely strange environment and I don't even know where the toilet is, I feel panic stricken...In fact the fear of the unfamiliar gets worse as I get older because I realise there is more potential for an accident...A white stick, a guide dog, they don't really compensate. The only thing that really compensates when you're blind is a genuine human guide...I've missed out on lots of educational opportunities because it's so stressful and the older I get the more unwilling I am to put myself through it.*

These quotations illustrate that the barriers that visually impaired people, and indeed all disabled people, face are inter-related and cannot be effectively dismantled in a piecemeal fashion; it is of little use making a venue accessible to disabled people, for example, if they are unable to reach it (see Zarb 1995a, Thompson 1997, Swain et al 1998). Borland and James state that:

> *Access to facilities is often regarded as one of the most straightforward areas to deal with, but access issues, for students with a range of disabilities, are extremely complex.* (1999: 99)

Owen Hutchinson et al (1998) provide a great deal of practical advice on the removal of barriers to visually impaired students in further and higher education, with regard to the immediate physical environment, and access to the curriculum including specialised technology, suitable lighting, colour contrast and modified assessment procedures. Curtis et al also provide advice on improving accessibility within venues for visually impaired students:

> *There are several principles to be followed if premises are to be easily accessible to visually impaired trainees. These include; good lighting, clear signs (print and braille) changing surface textures and white lines on stairs to give a few examples.* (1997: 11)

Problems of transport, mobility, teaching methods and staff attitudes and behaviour are noted in surveys of visually impaired students conducted by the RNIB (1996b. 1997) which conclude that all need to be improved.

Attitudes and Behaviour of Course Organisers and Fellow Students

Another barrier to inclusion which some of the physiotherapists highlighted was the attitudes and behaviour of course organisers and, sometimes, colleagues and fellow students. Hilary explained the problems she had had being accepted on to a course on manipulations:

> *They didn't give me reasons as an organisation but individuals in it made it very clear to me that they felt visually impaired people weren't able to manipulate. I made a very consistent, concerted effort over a number of years to maintain that that wasn't the case...They decided that entry to their two year course was by examination so if you passed the examination you were eligible for entry. So I put myself up for the examination and passed it and they had to offer me a place but they made it as difficult as possible for me to pass the examination. For example, they wouldn't provide me with the exam paper either on tape or in braille. They wouldn't provide me with a typewriter...They were very difficult but I was absolutely determined that I was going to do it.*

Eric experienced negative attitudes on a counselling course:

> *There was one tutor…and she had serious problems with blind people…she actually wrote in one of the counselling journals something like 'Although it is reasonable to allow a blind student to do the counselling course, if he or she has the qualifications, is it fair on the client to subject them to a blind counsellor?' I think it's outrageous…And some of the students on that course were very anti-blind people.*

These experiences not only highlight blatant discrimination but also illustrate how visual impairment is stigmatised (Goffman 1968) and embellished, according to time and culture, with social meaning (Hahn 1990, Swain and French 1998). There is a growing literature on the negative imagery of disabled people and the adverse effect that this can have on their lives (Barnes 1992, Pointon and Davies 1997, Cooke et al 2000). Blind people, for example, have frequently been depicted as burdens and as objects of pity (French and Swain 1997).

Julia was prevented from doing a paediatric course on the grounds of her visual impairment:

> *People say you can't work with children but that is rubbish because you always have a parent or a carer there. That was one of my arguments with the Bobath Centre, they wouldn't let me do the paediatric course years ago because they said silly things like 'How can you tell where the head is if you're holding the pelvis?'. Now I found it hard to explain to them how I could tell because obviously we didn't share the same experience. But you never have a child there without its mother who can tell you how they are responding. They can't make that leap of comprehension because they aren't you. They haven't got the experience of being blind from birth and having compensating strategies…I had a place funded to go on the paediatric Bobath course but the Bobath Centre wouldn't let me go on it. That has been the experience of several blind physios…It's taken years to change them.*

Jenny, Sandra and Sheila had similar experiences:

> *She said that due to the way they ran their courses, which was by lots of slides and visual demonstrations, that they could not see how I could do it. I said that she was treating me like a second class citizen but she said she was just being realistic…In the end she said she was prepared to let me come for a month, when there was no course going on, but I wouldn't get the qualification. I went along with that because I knew that I wasn't going to win and I needed the knowledge* (Jenny)

> *We had a new teacher who asked how he could help because he realised I couldn't see. I said 'Well you could give handouts of what you are going to put on the board' but he said he couldn't do that and he never asked again.* (Sandra)

There was a course advertised for using the gymnastic ball... I rang up... and she said 'I've already got a lot of people booked on the course and I don't think I could helpfully teach you in that group'. But she invited me to come along at another time when she would show me some things herself which she did. I went at the end of the afternoon and she gave me an hour of her time. It wasn't the same as going on the course but she didn't just say 'sorry I can't help you because you can't see/'.

Ash et al (1997) highlight the lack of knowledge and awareness of staff in mainstream colleges regarding disability and Borland and James (1999) believe that tutors usually think in terms of the medical model of disability, rather than the social model, and therefore react to students, at best, as people who need care rather than people who have rights.

Julia faced negative attitudes from other physiotherapists which nearly prevented her from doing a course on neurology:

Before we did the course itself, we did three weekends on normal movement which tended to be rather packed. I took one particular facilitator with me who tended to be a bit aggressive about people being considerate, getting in the way and whatever, and at the end of the course I heard that three out of 20 people said on their forms that having a visually impaired person on the course slowed it down...We were so angry, my facilitator and I, but my superintendent's attitude was 'Oh dear, we mustn't upset the people who are paying these vast fees' she said 'I can't put you on the course if people are expected to pay £800.' I wrote her a very firm and forceful letter and she said 'I bet if I refuse to let you go on it you'll say I'm discriminating' and I said 'Of course I'll say that, you won't dare do that.' In fact it worked out fine. I had a different facilitator who was much more tactful...I found that gradually the other members got used to me and I worked with different people and it was fine. It's always a bit of a gamble the first time.

Sheila faced more subtle negativity from one of her colleagues during in-service training:

Somebody had brought along a new kind of seating for the young chronic sick and my assistant thoughtfully took me to feel it. But another physiotherapist who was there was quite edgy about me going up to feel it again, about me being in people's way and that kind of thing. She was someone who I worked in the hospital with who I hadn't had any difficulty with, but I suddenly registered her embarrassment in front of other colleagues.

These quotations illustrate Goffman's notion of 'courtesy stigma' (Goffman 1968) whereby the stigma of an impairment can 'contaminate' those in proximity to it, in this case other members of the profession. It is stated in an RNIB survey of visually impaired students that:

> The evidence clearly suggests that the levels of awareness of the learning needs of visually impaired students are not always apparent and demonstrate major shortcomings particularly in more formal institutional settings. Teachers and lecturers, particularly in situations where visually impaired students are integrated into mainstream provision, when presented with the challenge of a blind or partially sighted student can become quickly overawed. (1996b: 30)

Feelings of Embarrassment and Anxiety

Some of the barriers the physiotherapists experienced gave rise to feelings of embarrassment and anxiety which could become barriers in themselves. As Owen Hutchinson et al state:

> Many blind and partially sighted people describe various psychological responses to specific situations which can be classified as secondary barriers. (1998: 93–4)

Sarah, for example, would not ask for help in front of lots of other people because she did not want to 'draw attention to herself'. Josephine expressed similar feelings and also worried that her presence might have an adverse effect on other course participants:

> I find it a bit embarrassing in a new setting…one never wishes to stand out somehow…They're mostly very nice to me, but I'm very keen not to block someone else's view or take the limelight. I don't like to be prominent.

Terry had similar feelings:

> For me, as a visually impaired person, there's still, not quite embarrassment – I was going to say humiliation but that's too strong as well – of having to get up from the group, walk to the front so you can see or feel what the person's doing…you think 'Here we go'. Maybe it's just my problem. You're different from everyone…I still struggle with that a bit.

Several physiotherapists found the social side of courses particularly problematic. Alice described the problem of coping with the buffet lunch:

> The business of even seeing what's on the board for lunch, I can't see the blessed board and I don't feel confident serving myself, I can't see what all the food is and the thought of carrying it to the table and crashing into somebody because I've got the most minute field of vision. That sort of thing is embarrassing, it's frightening and it thoroughly puts me off…You've got to explain to people the help you need and sometimes it's all too exhausting and I'm put off…Being blind is exhausting isn't it? You can never let go and relax unless you have somebody to really rely on.

These feelings of embarrassment and anxiety which are likely, at least in part, to be generated by the hostile physical and social environment, may contribute to the reluctance of some of the physiotherapists to ask for help. This is illustrated in the following quotations:

> *No I don't always ask, I must admit that, so I'm probably as much at fault. They have offered recently to give me a couple of the overheads but I've not bothered because I haven't got anyone to read them to me.* (Sheila)

> *The general in-service training, well they usually use overheads and things, but I never say 'Can I have printed copies?'. I usually try to get as much information as I can glean. I thought it was too much hassle to ask for information.* (Sarah)

Asking for help and giving explanations involves 'work' on the part of disabled people and may only partially solve the problem. This is recognised by the disabled people's movement which promotes collective action rather than individual action.

These feelings of inadequacy and embarrassment may be due, in part, to internal oppression whereby disabled people internalise the view that their needs are less important than those of the majority and that they are less worthy of consideration (Mason 1992, Woolley 1993, French 1993a, Oliver and Barnes 1998). It may also reflect the difficulty and ineffectiveness of trying to bring about change as isolated individuals and without strong legislative backing (Barnes 1991, Oliver 1990, 1996c). Baron et al, talking of disabled social work students, state that:

> *Once accepted, the students were reluctant to contact institutions about their needs prior to the start of the programme as they felt this might lead them to be labelled as a nuisance. Without the initiative being taken by the institution, this resulted in students entering a programme with no clear strategic plan of how to create the conditions which would allow them to meet its requirements.* (1996: 373)

McDonald (1996) considers that it is unwise and unjust to expect disabled students to be responsible for their own inclusion.

Although the physiotherapists were generally pleased with any assistance they received, many found it inadequate and tokenistic. Terry said:

> *It's the old, old story you know...With the best possible intentions people make a token gesture don't they? They send you a form which says 'Do you have any special needs?' you say 'Yes, I don't see very well' and their compromise is that they allocate you a seat at the front of the class and usually that's not enough because you still can't see the overheads...They often ask if you want copies of the overheads afterwards, which is nice, but it would be better if you had them at the time. It's tokenism as far as I'm concerned.*

He went on to explain that, in his experience, the only people who provide adequate help are other visually impaired people:

It tends to be very ad hoc the in-service training, it's usually done by a member of staff although they might invite someone over to do things. If it's an outside speaker they have never made any kind of effort for visually impaired people, if it's the inside staff sometimes people have made the effort, but the people who make the effort most are fellow visually impaired people. If they do the in-service training they will have taken the time to do large print hand-outs, to allocate seats at the front and they invite you to come up and get involved.

It is clear that the barriers the physiotherapists experienced lay at all three levels of the social model of disability and the SEAwall of institutional discrimination as discussed in chapter 1. The physiotherapists frequently encountered difficult and unthinking attitudes and behaviour, a hostile physical environment and difficulty managing within organisations whose norms and ethos were geared to non-disabled people. Being well known by colleagues did not automatically reduce these problems as might be expected.

Preece (1997) believes that provision for disabled students needs to occur on both an individual level and an institutional level. It appears that, in many instances, this was not occurring for the visually impaired physiotherapists. Leicester and Lovell, in their study of disabled students state:

It seemed to us that all our interviewees experienced socially imposed restrictions such that impairment is more disabling than it need be...the educational experiences of all those we interviewed suggest the urgent need for radical educational changes in Britain towards a more enabling education. (1997: 17–18)

This view is shared by the RNIB:

Visually impaired students...have yet to claim their full entitlement to educational opportunities. There is a clear and urgent need to raise levels of awareness within establishments generally and for programmes of development and training to be introduced for staff. Research is also required into what constitutes good practice within the field of teaching methodology. (1996b: 30)

Coping Strategies

Coping strategies have been defined by Gross as:

Conscious ways of trying to adapt to stress and anxiety in a positive and constructive way by using thoughts and behaviour orientated towards searching for information, problem solving, seeking help from others, recognising our true feelings and establishing goals and objectives. (1987: 445)

In relation to disabled people, Owen Hutchinson et al define coping strategies as:

...the means by which a disabled person seeks to take control over a given situation in order to be able to manage the environment, negative attitudes and poor practice. It is also, however, a means by which a person's own resources are utilised to make the most of any situation. (1998: 96)

Lazarus and Folkman (1984) distinguish between problem-focused coping strategies and emotion-focused coping strategies although they believe that the strategies are usually combined. Problem-focused coping may involve alterations to the external environment in order to solve a problem, for example replacing steps with a ramp for wheelchair users, or acquiring a new skill to cope with a particular situation. Emotion-based coping involves cognitive changes within the individual, for example deciding that an issue is no longer important. Defence mechanisms such as denial and suppression, as formulated by Freud, can also be viewed as emotion-focused coping strategies (Atkinson et al 1993). Avoidance of a problem is a further coping strategy which may be adopted (Ogden 1996).

The coping strategies chosen will depend upon the resources available to the individual, including social support and his or her degree of power, within a particular context, to affect change. The significance of the problem to the person, as well as the person's overall evaluation of the problem, is also important (Lazarus and Folkman 1984). Human beings show diversity in response to situations according to how they appraise them (Atkinson et al 1993). Information about the problem and past experience of dealing with similar problems may also influence the coping strategy adopted by the individual.

According to Lazarus and Folkman (1984), when people are confronted with a problem they firstly define it and then generate solutions to it. They then weigh up the alternative solutions, in terms of costs and benefits, and finally choose and implement a solution. Coping strategies which involve assertion and attempts to modify the environment are congruent with the social model of disability.

Owen Hutchenson et al (1998) describe various coping strategies which are used by visually impaired people. These may be cognitive, for example when a visually impaired person develops a good memory to compensate for lack of accessible information; sensory, for example when a visually impaired person concentrates on auditory cues to compensate for a lack of visual cues; or practical, as when a visually impaired person seeks assistance or learns a new skill to overcome, minimise or manage a problem. Coping strategies frequently cannot be implemented without some cost to the individual, for example taking longer over tasks, expending energy on adapting the environment, or avoiding difficult situations which it would be better, in the long run, to confront. The coping strategies used by the visually impaired physiotherapists will now be discussed.

Attending Courses with a Sighted Person

Some of the physiotherapists interviewed, particularly those who are totally blind, would only attend courses if they were accompanied by a sighted person. It has already been noted that Alice takes her husband and Julia uses a facilitator. Julia explained:

> *The happiest conclusion I've come to in the last five years, mainly because I've become less worried about being 'normal', is that I've started to approach course organisers to have a facilitator...I've found that when I've asked the Chartered Society, the Disabled Living Foundation, the Learning Disabilities Association, they have all said that I can bring someone along free of charge to facilitate me. It's worked out beautifully.*

Julia brings up the issue of normality and the pressures disabled people feel to 'fit in' to the norm. Baron et al (1996) believe that teaching practices are often subconsciously based upon assumptions of normality which render them very resistant to change. They found that:

> *Where teaching staff did bring such issues to consciousness and take enabling action, it tended to be for a brief interlude before old recipes reasserted themselves and exclusion resumed.* (1996: 372)

Owen Hutchinson et al believe that:

> *Within the medical model it is axiomatic that an individual is expected to 'cope' with disability regardless of the cost to that person. Success is judged by criteria that presuppose that 'normality' is a desirable state.* (1998: 94)

Sarah attends courses with a sighted person but does not find that it solves all the problems:

> *I always manage to go with somebody, but even then, even your sighted colleagues who work with you all the time, don't understand that you miss out so much not being able to see the overheads and the demonstrations.*

Malcolm likes to have a sighted person with him but if this is not possible he is undeterred. He said '...sometimes I just have to bowl in and hope for the best'. Hilary is also prepared to attend courses alone but recognises the necessity to be assertive:

> *It can be a problem to get from a to b, to find the place, but I'm quite out-going in the sense that if I don't know I'll ask...if I arrive in a room full of strangers who are all helping themselves to coffee I'll just ask someone to get me some. There's usually someone there who will help.*

Being Proactive and Assertive

Some of the physiotherapists were sufficiently proactive and assertive to explain their particular needs to course organisers. The results of this are, however, variable. Ben related his experiences on an M.Sc course in the early 1990s:

> *Some people were excellent, they transferred all their overheads into handouts for me and I was able to follow it perfectly. Other people, probably ones who were slightly more removed from the immediate course team, made no concessions at all...I just had to manage the best I could. Of course my fellow course members were helpful, telling me what the board said and things like that if I needed it. It went from one extreme to the other.*

Problems of access for disabled students in universities is well recognised (Wolfendale and Corbett 1996). A survey by the RNIB (1998) found access within colleges poor for visually impaired people although the numbers of visually impaired students in further and higher education has steadily increased (Simkiss et al 1998).

A few physiotherapists were prepared to challenge lecturers directly if their needs were not met. John said:

> *There's quite a trend with lecturers to say 'Do this' and 'Do that' and one thing you can do as a physiotherapist is use accurate terminology...With things like that I've got a bit more pushy, I say 'Excuse me, can you be a bit more precise with your descriptions and anatomical terms?'.*

Some of the physiotherapists telephone or write to course organisers in advance to explain their needs. The results of this are, however, variable and rarely straightforward as the following quotations illustrates:

> *I've arranged to have print or braille stuff in advance. I think that people on the whole, if you approach them in the right way, are pretty helpful. You have to ask but it's not so much that they don't want to help, they just don't think about it, they just forget.* (Malcolm)

> *Very often I would ask for things in advance and sometimes I would get them and sometimes not, it was pretty haphazard. My guess is that people might be a bit more aware of it now.* (Robert)

It can be seen from these quotations that being proactive and assertive may be helpful but does not necessarily bring about the desired result. Cost can be used as a convenient excuse although adaptations for visually impaired people, for example copying overhead projector slides, are not necessarily expensive. Cost can, however, be an issue when attempting to include disabled students in mainstream education as noted by Preece:

> *...the cost of supporting disabled people conflicts with competitive market-tied funding policies. The disabled student becomes an economically expensive, and therefore potentially undesirable, per capita commodity.* (1995: 98)

Avoidance and the Use of 'Special' Courses

A minority of the physiotherapists avoided courses altogether because of the barriers they posed and some used the strategy of attending, primarily or exclusively, courses run by the ABCP (now the AVICP). John said:

> *The nice thing about the ABCP is that, with the courses that are organised there, you know that things are going to be set up for you. I go to quite a few of those.*

The problem with this strategy is that it radically reduces choice. The AVICP can only run courses which will attract considerable numbers so physiotherapists who work in minority specialities, such as psychiatry and learning difficulties, are not well served.

Spontaneous Help

In some instances substantial help is provided spontaneously and some of the physiotherapists were forced to rely on this. Hilary recalled how she was helped by fellow students on a demanding professional course on manipulations:

> *They were extremely helpful because there was a vast quantity of reading material that had to be done in a short space of time. I used the Express Reading Service (a tape reading service run by the RNIB) for lots of it but the volume was virtually unmanageable for sighted people so what they did in the second year of the course, when we were all bogged down, they actually split the reading material between them and reviewed it for me and presented me with the abstracts which was quite unbelievable.*

Some of the physiotherapists did rely, at least in part, on luck, for example help from other students, as a mechanism for getting through courses. It is noted by Baron et al (1996), when talking of social work education, however, that the help disabled students receive from other students tends to fall away when academic pressure becomes high. It can also be argued that the system is at fault if disabled students are forced to rely on other students for assistance.

It can be seen from this account that the visually impaired physiotherapists use a variety of coping strategies to overcome or minimise the barriers they encounter in post-registration education. These include arranging and accepting help from others, being proactive and assertive, and avoiding difficult situations. Barnes (1996) highlights three coping strategies that he has used as a visually impaired person both at college and at work: minimisation (playing down the problems and trying to appear 'normal'); compensation (trying to perform at a higher standard than others); and openness (being open and assertive about disability). Similar strategies have been described by Goffman (1968). The visually impaired physiotherapists used all of these strategies, as well as avoidance, with regard to post-registration education but were predominantly proactive and assertive.

Physiotherapists' Views of Integrated Education for Visually Impaired Physiotherapists

The North London School of Physiotherapy for the Visually Handicapped closed in 1995 between the first and second phases of the study. The visually impaired physiotherapists had mixed views about the closure of this facility and the inclusion of visually impaired physiotherapy students in mainstream universities. Some people looked back at their struggles in integrated education. Lucy said:

> *When I first heard that the school was closing I did write saying I was concerned about the support the students would get...I personally started my training at an ordinary physiotherapy school and transferred to the RNIB school because I didn't get the support.*

Another physiotherapist, Sandra, had discontinued her studies of physiotherapy at a mainstream college, through lack of support, and re-trained at the RNIB physiotherapy college some time later.

Terry's views on the inclusion of visually impaired physiotherapy students were influenced by his experience of mainstream education as a child:

> Yes, I did regret the closure of the school because I thought it was a dedicated unit specifically for people with visual impairments and I'm a product of somebody whose been through the system, whose done OK out of it, so I know there will be people who will struggle...I went to ordinary secondary school but I just couldn't manage...I didn't get any qualifications, got no specialist help, I had a very bad experience of integration. I've got a twin brother and I just used to sit there and copy his notes, that's all I could do. My school reports all used to say 'Terry's a good student, he tries very hard, but is seriously held back by his eye sight problem' but nobody ever said 'Why don't you go somewhere else?'...I didn't even know that there were such places. I went to the special college in Hereford for three years when I was 19 to do my 'O' and 'A' levels and then I went to physio college. It's the best thing that ever happened to me...being with other visually impaired people felt perfectly all right.

Charlotte, who also went through mainstream education, had similar feelings:

> ...I benefited by going to the RNIB School. My sight had always been made light of and probably, rather than admitting that I needed help, I would have glossed over and muddled through if you like. Whereas, because everything was geared to us there, there were no gaps.

Stephen spoke of the benefits for him of being with other visually impaired people:

> When you come back from your first encounter with a ward you can say to the other students 'I had a hell of a day today!'...people can support you in your 'down' days and you start to learn from one another how to cope; whether there is some kind of tactile cue on the floor, how you go about chatting up the Sister to get information about the patients...it's what I call experiential learning in a practical way. I didn't feel at all odd. Now once you get out into the world you are, of course, odd because you are different, but at least by that time you have been taught by your peers, who have been before you, or with you, and you can learn from one another. You have a foundation for coping.

Curtis et al (1997) stress the importance of disabled people establishing a shared identity with others in a similar situation in today's climate of integration.

Some of the physiotherapists had met visually impaired physiotherapy students who had come to work in their hospitals or units on clinical placements. Andrea said:

> I find it very difficult to believe that they can manage in an integrated situation. I mean we had one of the partially sighted students last year...I was asked to have a talk with her because she was struggling so much. And that was someone

who could read but she was really having a hard time of it and she was thinking about giving it up...I don't think I would do it now if I had my choice again. But yet, having said that, I suppose the younger people coming through are used to computers and, of course, I'm not. So from that point of view it might be easier for them.

Simkiss et al (1998) found that visually impaired pupils and students perform equally well on examinations whether or not they are in mainstream or specialised settings. They found that the visually impaired people they interviewed were equally negative about mainstream and special schools. They state:

Evidence from the focus groups indicate that mainstream provision may need to develop greater awareness of the requirements of visually impaired students and expertise in meeting their requirements, whilst specialist provision may need to take care to avoid over-protectiveness and to encourage external links. (1998: 12)

Some physiotherapists felt that the closure of the special physiotherapy college heralded the end of physiotherapy as a career for totally blind people and perhaps all visually impaired people. This view was voiced most strongly by totally blind physiotherapists themselves. Stephen said:

I think that totally blind people will not be trained anymore. I think it's a profession that is shut to totally blind people and I think that is a disgrace...I would love to be proved wrong, I really would, but I can't see a totally blind student going through mainstream physiotherapy training. I don't think it would be possible at all.

Some of the physiotherapists regarded the competition which visually impaired people would experience when applying for a place on a mainstream physiotherapy course as a potentially serious barrier. Pam said:

I think at that school they took people who weren't really 'A' students. I don't know whether anyone will continue to do that now...I don't know how well we will compete with all these high-flyers – I expect some people will.

Few of the physiotherapists were surprised by the closure of the special college and many speculated upon the reasons for its demise. Malcolm foresaw the closure of the college, and is doubtful that totally blind people will train as physiotherapists again. He is conscious, however that his thoughts may be filtered through his perceptions as an older person:

It saddened me I think but, on the other hand, I was talking to someone ten years before and we decided between us that it wouldn't last. The numbers of totally blind young people are dropping so the need for the school lessened. Not that I'm saying that partially sighted folk don't need assistance, but it was the totally blind students I think that really kept that college going, certainly in the earlier years. I foresee very few totally blind people going into physio in the future. There are fewer that will achieve the right academic standard. I think the system has changed so that they would find it very stressful to do it. I would never say that a 'total' can't do it but they are going to have to be incredibly well motivated...But then I'm looking at it from an older person's point of view...20 years ago I might have been saying 'No problem at all, let's go and do it, fine'.

Malcolm also believes that the special college may have deterred people with some sight from applying and that their numbers in the profession may, conversely, increase if mainstream colleges are willing to accept them:

It would seem to be that there are quite a few (partially sighted people) applying. I think there might be more because they're not in the environment of having to work with the totally blind. Now there was only ever one chap who actually made a comment about that during our training and he said 'Having 'totals' around restrains what we can do' and he wasn't being nasty, he was making what I regarded as a sensible comment. People coming from mainstream school found it really strange to go there.

I have noted that during my training at the RNIB School of Physiotherapy from 1968 to 1972, I was, for the first time treated more as a blind person than a partially sighted person which I did, indeed, find strange even though I had been through special education for partially sighted children:

Although about half the students were partially sighted, one of the criteria for entry to the college was the ability to read and write braille (which I had never used before) and to type proficiently as, regardless of the clarity of their handwriting, the partially sighted students were not permitted to write their essays or examinations by hand...No visual teaching methods were used in the college and, for those of us with sight, it was no easy matter learning subjects like anatomy, physiology and biomechanics without the use of diagrams. (French 1993a: 75)

This situation changed over the years but is, nonetheless, confirmed in the 1981 promotional literature of NLSP where it is stated:

No difference is made between students who are totally blind and those with some degree of residual vision. All training is based on totally blind techniques. This is essential as, even with a stable prognosis, provision must be made for eventual function as a blind person. It is also a fact that many partially sighted

> *students think they can see more than they can; their accuracy is improved when they accept a 'blind' technique...a degree of vision should only be regarded as a bonus.* (1981: 10)

This patronising and oppressive treatment of visually impaired students with some sight may have helped to justify the existence of the special college by exaggerating the differences between them and sighted physiotherapy students.

Eric spoke about the economic reason for the closure of the college and speculated on whether people had already decided that physiotherapy was no longer a suitable profession for blind people long before the special college was closed:

> *I was very saddened that it closed but I understand the reasons – financial and the number of students was just too small. I wonder too, though it was never said, whether people had come to the conclusion that physiotherapy was not possible for blind people anymore. I think it was inevitable with the amount the RNIB was subsidising the school, it was getting on for three quarters of a million per year with just a handful of UK students.*

At the time of the closure of the physiotherapy college in 1995 it had been affiliated to the City University in London for six years. Some of the physiotherapists had hoped that it might have survived by accepting sighted physiotherapy students. Pam said:

> *I thought 'Why can't they integrate fully sighted people with us?', to integrate that way round...I think they said that they couldn't because of the RNIB – for whatever reason it couldn't be done.*

Many of the physiotherapists spoke about the necessity of specialised teaching methods and equipment and were doubtful or uncertain about whether they would be provided on a mainstream course. Julia said:

> *I think it will put off totally blind people from training and I can't imagine how they can have the same quality of practical skills training. I think it's slower for us to learn practical skills than sighted people. I can't see how they can cope on equal terms.*

Terry, on the other hand, felt optimistic about inclusion provided the necessary support was provided.

Sharron found the special college rather insular and did not regret its demise. She was, however, uncertain about whether educational inclusion would work:

I think it's a good thing that it closed down. The problem was that there was only one institution of its kind, so it was very dependent on the staff and the quality of teaching that was there...on the face of it we can say that integration is a good thing but not having personal knowledge of people who have been through the system it's very difficult to say whether it's better.

As noted in chapter 4, in 1998 16 visually impaired physiotherapists were enrolled in mainstream physiotherapy courses including four totally blind students. The views of many of the visually impaired physiotherapists regarding the recruitment of totally blind candidates may, therefore, be unduly pessimistic although the numbers are very small. The situation needs to be carefully monitored.

Conclusion

In this chapter data from the 20 interviews undertaken in the second phase of the study have been analysed to examine the experiences of visually impaired physiotherapists in relation to their inclusion in post-registration education, and their views concerning the inclusion of visually impaired people in mainstream physiotherapy education. The chapter has highlighted the numerous barriers to educational inclusion that visually impaired physiotherapists experience and the strategies they use to overcome, minimise or manage them. These barriers are largely the same as those reported in the first phase of the study despite the implementation of equal opportunity policies and the Disability Discrimination Act (1995). This Act is, however, extremely weak particularly with regard to education. Education which occurs at work, for example in-service training, is, however, covered by that part of the Act which relates to employment (see chapter 2) so inadequate work-based education does contravene the Act.

Most of the barriers the physiotherapists experienced can be placed within the context of the social model of disability and institutional discrimination. The physiotherapists experienced attitudinal, environmental and structural barriers in their attempts to be included in post-registration education. These barriers were wide-ranging, involving not only lack of access to learning materials, but problems with travel and mobility within unfamiliar environments and the speed at which activities are undertaken. Many, although not all, of the instances of blatant attitudinal discrimination had occurred many years ago, but lack of adequate provision and assistance and covert attitudinal discrimination were still evident.

The visually impaired physiotherapists talked about personal feelings of, for example, embarrassment which, though frequently resulting from other people's behaviour and the disabling physical environment could become barriers in themselves. Such 'internal' or psychological barriers are spoken of less frequently within the context of the social model of disability and institutional discrimination than the more tangible external barriers. The absence of theorising at the level of the disabled individual within the social model of disability has not, however, gone unnoticed particularly by disabled women (see Crow 1996, Morris 1996) who have sought to extend the social model of disability by focusing on the individual as well as on the external environment (see chapter 1).

This analysis shows that educational barriers differ according to the degree of impairment; totally blind people, for example, experience more difficulty with travel and negotiating unfamiliar environments than people with some sight. Some of the physiotherapists also indicated that the barriers were related, at least in part, to their age. It is not clear why this should be so but it may be the case that, with the normal decline of hearing as people get older, mobility becomes more difficult particularly for totally blind physiotherapists who are sometimes dependent on echo location (the detection of objects through changes in sound) when moving about. It may also be the case, as Andrea said, that some of the older physiotherapists are not experienced with the latest technology which may assist with administrative tasks. The effects of age and the level of impairment on the barriers encountered is rarely discussed within the framework of the social model of disability and deserves further study.

The physiotherapists used a variety of coping strategies to overcome, minimise or manage the barriers they experienced. These were frequently geared towards changing the external environment, for example taking a facilitator on courses or asking for the course materials to be provided in a suitable format. For such arrangements to occur it was necessary for the physiotherapists to be proactive and assertive. These problem-solving strategies, which are geared towards changing the external environment, fit with the tenets of the social model of disability, although it is recognised within the social model of disability that solving disabling barriers should not fall upon individual disabled people.

Some physiotherapists did, however, take a more passive stance of relying on spontaneous help or avoiding difficult situations altogether. Such behaviour is not irrational. The near impossibility of breaking down institutional disablism as an isolated individual, and the need for collective action, is well recognised within the disability literature (see Campbell and Oliver 1996). It is also clear from this account that being assertive and attempting to change the environment does not always succeed and can be exhausting. Taking a passive stance and avoiding difficult situations can thus be viewed as rational behaviour and may, in itself, be an assertive act.

In the eight year period between the first and second phases of the study, the special physiotherapy college for visually impaired students closed and the future of visually impaired physiotherapists has been left uncertain. The views of visually impaired physiotherapists, concerning inclusion in mainstream physiotherapy courses, are mixed and similar to the views expressed in the first phase of the study. Concern and scepticism were voiced about the continuing acceptance of totally blind candidates, particularly by totally blind physiotherapists themselves. Some of the physiotherapists were conscious, however, that their views may be coloured by their age and that younger visually impaired people are likely to have had different experiences, for example familiarity with technology, which may help them to overcome some of the barriers they encounter. It was noted in chapter 4 that totally blind people are now being educated as physiotherapists within mainstream universities.

The following chapter will examine the barriers the 20 physiotherapists, who were interviewed in the second phase of the study, encountered at work and the strategies they used to overcome, minimise or manage them. It will be noted how far their situation has changed since the first phase of the study was undertaken.

Chapter 7

Employment: Barriers a Coping Strategies

This chapter will explore the barriers experienced by visually impaired physiotherapists at work and the strategies they adopt to overcome, minimise or manage them. The data will be drawn from the 20 interviews with visually impaired physiotherapists conducted in the second phase of the study. The physiotherapists encountered numerous barriers which are remarkably similar to those encountered by the visually impaired physiotherapists interviewed in the first phase of the study (see chapter 5) and broadly similar to those faced by other visually impaired people (Simkiss et al 1998) and disabled people at work (Barnes et al 1998, Burchardt 2000).

The physiotherapists experienced six significant barriers in their work: transport, therapeutic equipment, administration, the physical environment (particularly of wards), meetings and the attitudes and behaviour of colleagues and employers. These barriers, together with the strategies used to overcome, minimise or manage them, will each be considered in turn.

Transport

Barriers

Thirteen of the 20 physiotherapists mentioned lack of personal transport as a problem in their working lives. Pam felt compelled to work in areas with good public transport:

> *I would love to be able to just take off...But it's a problem when you want to change jobs. I was thinking I'd like to go to Harrogate, it would be beautiful country side...they told me they had three hospitals that were 11 miles apart, I didn't apply...You need to stay in the city or to go somewhere where the transport is good.*

Limited public transport prevented some physiotherapists from working in specialities of their choice. Jenny explained:

...hen I was at the senior 2 level I worked with amputees, and really enjoyed that, but decided that in terms of specialising...most of the specialist amputee units are on sites that are either too far away geographically or they are not accessible by public transport.

The physiotherapists who worked in the community faced particular problems with travel. Terry described how he travels around London to reach clients' homes:

It means I have to go everywhere by bus. The problem is I have to deliver frames, so I sometimes have to get on a bus with a walking frame...I try and avoid it when the kids are going to school, or coming home from school, or in the rush hour...I've managed it so far. If I get really desperate, like if I have a really big piece of equipment to take, then I'll tell the manager and she'll arrange for me to go round in a cab and drop it off.

Some people felt that the increase in community work was creating a growing problem for visually impaired physiotherapists. Lucy said:

I think this (travelling) is a problem for visually impaired physios working in the rehab field, because home visiting is becoming a bigger thing and you can't do that. Jobs that require a lot of home visiting are really out because you have to be able to drive. In a rural area like this there is no way you can do it unless you can drive.

Hilary, who was relocated to a new post against her will, found the Hospital Trust very unsympathetic to the transport problems she faced:

I was relocated to another hospital which was extremely difficult for me to get to from home. It required catching three buses. So I actually had to take out a grievance with the Trust about it...the Access to Work people supported me partially to help me with taxi fares home. I walked in the morning, and it was over three miles, but I got a taxi home in the evening.

Sheila believes that much of the problem arises because the ability to drive has become the norm:

Very many physios have transport of their own whereas when I first qualified that wasn't the case, a lot of physios travelled around on public transport, as I did, but now times have changed...it's become the norm and, depending on your job, that is another difference to be overcome.

The problems of transport for a wide range of disabled people, including visually impaired people, have been widely documented (RADAR 1990, Barnes 1991, French 1993b, French and Swain 1997, RNIB 1998). It was noted in chapter 5 that fewer visually impaired physiotherapists, when compared with sighted physiotherapists, work in the community and that transport was raised as a problem. Heiser states that '…most of the journeys people make in this country are journeys that disabled people find problematical or impossible' (1995: 52) and Burchardt (2000) found that access to a car is associated with a better chance of being in work. This illustrates how the wider infrastructure affects the ability of disabled people to work and to do work of their choice.

Strategies

A variety of coping strategies were used to overcome, minimise or manage these transport problems. Sheila received help from the Access to Work scheme (see chapter 2) as well as from colleagues during a difficult period:

> *Through Access to Work I was granted help to meet the cost of a taxi to take me to work. It was granted to me because there was lots of building machinery in the area and it would have been far too dangerous for me to go into the hospital alone…That was the first time I had ever had help with transport to my work.*

Ben, who is a physiotherapy lecturer, visits students on their clinical placements, in various hospitals and centres, as part of his role. He is helped with this by considerate colleagues:

> *Fortunately it seems to be the policy that you go back mostly to the same places each time which is sensible for everyone. They've also given me places to visit with which I've had connections, or ones which are reasonably easy to get to by public transport, so I don't find it too bad.*

Sharron, who works in the community uses public transport, or she walks, but she can use taxis some of the time, although this gives rise to feelings of guilt:

> *If it's difficult to get to I can get a cab and the hospital pays, also if I have to take out large pieces of equipment I get a cab…But I always think about the money element – you know how much more is it costing if I get a cab to see someone compared with my colleagues who go by car? On the other hand, there are other staff in the hospital who regularly use cabs and don't seem to be bothered about the financial side of things at all!*

Stephen has been provided with a car by the Hospital Trust and is driven to appointments by a physiotherapy assistant:

> *The Trust has put at my disposal a car which I use for business mileage...it does mean that if I have to go to say...well I had to go to Leeds to sit on the NHS Equal Opportunities Working Party and because it is such a nightmare to get to Leeds on the train...the assistant actually drives me there.*

John and Josephine, who are both guide dog users, prefer to live sufficiently near work to walk. John said:

> *I now live about two and a half miles from the hospital and I walk it both ways. There's a bus service but I hate waiting for buses. To that end I've got a guide dog.*

A variety of strategies were used by the physiotherapists to overcome, minimise or manage transport barriers including the use of the Access to Work scheme, negotiation with managers, and personal strategies such as living near the work place and walking to work. The physiotherapists were treated in many different ways by the Hospital Trusts with one person having to walk to work and another being provided with a car. These two people are both managers, though the person provided with the car is a senior manager which may have accounted for his more favourable treatment. Many of the physiotherapists were left with a considerable degree of personal struggle over travel and lack of choice regarding employment. Some people, in addition, felt guilty about receiving assistance.

Therapeutic Equipment

Barriers

Six of the physiotherapists mentioned problems with using therapeutic equipment. Equipment was a particular problem in out-patient settings. Malcolm, who works in an out-patient department, explained the problem:

> *There's some stuff around nowadays that is not easy to use. I bung bits of 'high-mark' (a tactile marking substance) on which does work on the whole. One interferential machine we've got is not easy to use. In fact as a totally blind person, or a non-display reading person, you wouldn't be able to use it. But there is an older one that I can use...You can still find stuff but you have to look around...They're using more visual displays and it's all computerised, it's very flat, you don't have the landmarks that you used to have, there's the touch-sensitive keyboard thing. It's the way everything has gone, if you look throughout domestic appliances it's the same.*

Strategies

In physiotherapy practice clinicians have autonomy to choose which therapeutic interventions to use; in this way they may be at an advantage when compared with disabled people in non-professional jobs. Many of the physiotherapists could avoid equipment which posed particular problems for them. Hilary and John, who both work in out-patient departments, are unimpressed with the research evidence for the use of electrotherapy and choose not to use it very much. John said:

> *I'm not an electrotherapy person, I use TENS (trans-electrical nerve stimulation) and I use interferential. There is an ultra-sound/interferential combined unit which I can't use…I don't know whether it's impossible to use it as a blind person but because I'm very disenchanted with ultra-sound I've no great desire to learn how to use it. And with lasers, well reading all the research, it's very doubtful whether it's of any benefit whatsoever…Equipment hasn't really been an issue.*

Many of the physiotherapists worked in areas where electrotherapy equipment is used very little. Terry, who works in the field of psychiatry, said '…It's not really a high-tech environment…we don't have a lot of things with flashing lights.' One of the advantages of physiotherapy as a job for visually impaired people is its great diversity which allows difficulties to be avoided.

Sarah uses the older models of equipment as far as possible and asks the patients to help if she cannot manage:

> *There's one ultra-sound that I can use except that I can't see how many minutes are coming into the box and I just get the patients to tell me…the patients don't mind at all if you say, 'can you tell me when the needle gets to 2?'.*

Other physiotherapists are assisted by colleagues. Andrea said:

> *When I was in out-patients the other physios seemed to be quite able and capable and willing to mark things like timers and settings on dials for me…We either did it with little bits of sticky plaster or 'high-marks'.*

In the early days of visually impaired people practising physiotherapy, some of the manufacturers incorporated features into the electrotherapy machines specifically for visually impaired physiotherapists. Malcolm explained:

> *The EMS stuff is still quite good because they've taken an interest in us and I think Duffield have also incorporated audio stuff into their equipment…I think we were just in the right place at the right time…were you to try and do it now – no way.*

It is highly unusual for manufacturers to incorporate features into mainstream equipment to enable disabled people to use it. Disabled people are expected to use 'special' equipment which is usually more expensive, not widely available and more difficult to get repaired (Roulstone 1998).

Administration

Barriers

Nineteen of the 20 physiotherapists mentioned some degree of difficulty with administration the volume of which most people felt had increased over the years especially since the passing of the NHS and Community Care Act (1990). It was, however, also mentioned as a major barrier by the visually impaired physiotherapists in the first phase of the study before the Act was passed (see chapter 5). Andrea, who is totally blind, feels overwhelmed by paper work. This has led her to be less independent at work and less satisfied with it than she used to be:

> *It's a real problem...I'm told that I probably could cope with it on a computer but it's forms with little boxes which have to be ticked and it would be very difficult to set up I think...I suppose the answer is that I should keep more stuff in braille but it would take up so much room. I find it really difficult that everything that we plan...is all in print and there's no way I can go and look it up quickly...I sometimes sit there and think 'God, if only I could help the girls do some of it', work out some of the statistics or whatever we've got to do...When you get to the stage of thinking 'How many more years before I can retire?', just because you feel pressured, it's awful really. I don't think I would feel like that if work was how it used to be.*

Some of the physiotherapists could manage the administration but they found it time-consuming and a physical strain. Pam said:

> *I do the minimum...I have to get so close to the paper really. The older you get the more tension and back ache and neck ache you get leaning forward in awkward positions. Don't you find that?...I don't always record what I'm doing. If I've just taken someone for a little walk down the ward I might not log that...We have to record what we do though or they might think 'You're not working enough, we don't need you'.*

Terry and Lucy also experience physical symptoms which are brought on by reading print. Terry explained:

> *I can read ordinary sized print but it's very stressful and I've started to get this flashing that goes in front of my eyes and I get all these black dots that go across my vision. So it's hard work and I can't do it for long. Just recently I've started to get headaches, the last year or two, so I have to limit how much time I spend doing it. Where possible I try to get things in large print.*

Sarah finds that the thoughtless actions of colleagues makes the situation with administration more difficult:

> *I've always found this, wherever I've worked, that people always put memos on your desk and just leave them there…to me it's quite ridiculous to plonk a sighted memo on a blind person's desk and not explain what it's all about or reading it…I don't think it's a deliberate thing on their part and maybe because I don't make a fuss about it then…*

Accessibility of information is a major problem for visually impaired people (French and Swain 1997, Owen Hutchinson et al 1998, RNIB 1998) and many other disabled people (Barnes 1991, Parr et al 1997, Downs 1999). The physiotherapists experienced total or partial inaccessibility to the information they needed which was sometimes exacerbated by the behaviour of colleagues. Even the physiotherapists who could cope with administration were slow and tended to experience unpleasant physical symptoms from reading print such as headaches. This indicates the complexity of barrier removal – simply providing large print, for example, does not necessarily remove the barrier entirely.

Strategies

Readers Eleven of the 20 physiotherapists had readers paid for by the Access to Work scheme. The maximum number of hours allowed under this scheme is 15 per week. Stephen, who is a manager, has ten hours of reading assistance each week and Hilary has five. Sheila found a reader essential when she worked 'sole-charge' in a small hospital:

> *I had to arrange for my reader to come into the hospital to read me the notes of the patients because they were new to me and I had to deduce from the notes what I needed to know and make braille records of them, that's how I coped there. I was lucky that I had a reader who was actually able to come into the hospital to read to me because, obviously, I wouldn't be able to take the patients' notes outside the hospital.*

Some of the physiotherapists found using readers difficult for a variety of reasons. Hilary, who is a manager, found it hard to fit them in at times when she needed them most and found it best to use a variety of people and a variety of methods:

> *The problem is that I find it quite hard to use them during my working day...Sometimes it's possible to save things up and have them read at a later date but then at the moment when you have arranged for the person to come there's a crisis in the department that has to be dealt with...I use it very flexibly, what I often do is to have someone to read on to tape for me, and then sometimes I have someone to come in and do filing for me. I use different people. Sometimes I have someone to put stuff on to the computer for me so that I can read it through the voice synthesiser.*

Some physiotherapists had stopped using readers as, for various reasons, it had not worked well for them or other solutions had been found. Ben used a reader to read students' examination scripts and essays but found he did not concentrate very well. He now prefers to use a close circuit television which enlarges print:

> *I arranged to get one (a reader) through the Access to Work scheme...but she wasn't terribly good, I expect with practice she would have got better, but I decided it wasn't really worth it...With the best will in the world with readers it's sometimes difficult to concentrate hard enough, it's much better if you can read it yourself...So I've gone beyond readers. I'm pleased about it because I'm more versatile.*

The account the physiotherapists give of using readers illustrates that the removal of barriers is not easy. Reading aloud takes longer than reading to oneself and fitting readers into a busy and unpredictable working day is problematic.

Alternative equipment Most of the physiotherapists used alternative equipment to assist them with administrative tasks. This ranged from braille writing machines, powerful magnifying glasses, tape recorders and typewriters, to sophisticated computer equipment, braille printers and scanners (to read print aloud). For some physiotherapists the development of specialised computer software had made an enormous difference to their working lives. Terry, who uses a print enhancement system, said:

> *My world changed the day I got a computer. Really, I can't tell you, it's the most revolutionary thing that has happened to me since I've been a physio...I've always had problems with notes, every job I've ever been in nobody could read my hand-writing. I used to use a typewriter and then I applied to get a computer from the Access to Work scheme and I got given some training and, believe me, it's the best thing that ever happened to me. When I heard that the Government is changing the rules making the employers pay, Oh God! I've written to MPs*

over this because of the difference it's made to me...I flash it all up on the screen, all my patients' notes, current and from years gone by, large as I want. I can also print things out in large print so I can read it back.

Some of the physiotherapists, in contrast, resisted the use of computers and sophisticated equipment and preferred to use their current methods. Sarah said:

> I still use a manual typewriter...I suppose I find that so far I've got by, and I suppose this is why I've never pushed for the Access to Work scheme...I cope with my little methods with the bit of sight I've got...I'm so glad I can get by without learning all this new technology.

Others had found advice about the new equipment inadequate. Charlotte said:

> To start with it was like a nightmare really. I wouldn't have known about it except for my contact with Stephen...I didn't find them (Access to Work staff) at all helpful, they kept saying to me 'Well, what do you want?'. Well apart from talking to Robert and Stephen I didn't know what I wanted, I didn't know what the potential was...I actually wrote and complained...They brought the wrong thing three or four times and all that sort of thing. I find now that basically I don't have anything to do with them.

Other physiotherapists found the training inadequate. Julia explained:

> In 1991 I started to ask for equipment but I was so ignorant that I didn't really know what I needed and what was available. They supplied me with a lap-top computer which I found really difficult to learn because I had never had any computer training at all and just the concepts of word-processing were totally new and they wondered why I couldn't do it after two days training...They don't seem to realise that for a totally blind person learning any new piece of equipment is much harder.

Forty of the 55 visually impaired employees interviewed by Simkiss et al (1998) had technical equipment supplied through the Access to Work scheme to assist them at work. They too highlighted problems regarding insufficient training and delays in receiving the equipment – 12 waited more than three months and only seven received it within a month.

Malcolm and Stephen are largely self-taught even though the systems they use are more complicated than standard packages. Malcolm said:

> I basically taught myself...I'm interested in computing so it doesn't alarm me like it does some people. It wasn't too difficult...I spent quite a bit of my own time on it, learning how to use it and searching around for new information...I

had very little training but it didn't bother me a lot...But, on the other hand, it did take time. There should be sufficient training and there isn't.

Talking of visually impaired employees who use computer equipment, Simkiss et al state that '...most people had come to rely on their own resourcefulness and research skills to keep up to date' (1998: 111).

Employers are now asked to pay some of the cost of the equipment and services provided through the Access to Work scheme (Roulstone 1998). This is justified in the Disability Discrimination Act as employers are expected to take an active part in making employment accessible to disabled people (Doyle 1996). Many of the physiotherapists were alarmed and angry about this development. Stephen and Julia felt so strongly that they asked their employers not to contribute to the cost:

> *I've actually fought tooth and nail over the employers' contribution because I think it's a disadvantage and a disincentive for the employment of disabled people...I actually wrote to my employer and asked them not to support me in that sense which was a bit risky but I felt that was the way to get round it because I'm vehemently against that part of the employment scheme. OK this equipment is expensive, but if you were unemployed you would be costing the government a lot more. The equipment is sturdy...it can last for years.* (Stephen)

> *I wrote to personnel and said 'Please don't buy it for me'. But they did buy it...I could see they were being kind to me, they were trying to make me feel valued, but they were doing the worst possible thing regarding the legal rights of blind employees.* (Julia)

The ways in which technology can enhance the working lives of disabled people was considered in chapter 2. It was also noted, however, that technology has been used in an attempt to 'normalise' disabled people and 'correct' impairment. An individual, deficit model of disability has been adopted which views technology as a technical matter rather than a socio-political matter. Technology can become disabling if it is provided within a disabling environment.

Taking more time Twelve of the 20 physiotherapists said that they worked longer hours in order to hold down their jobs and this was particularly applicable to administration. The slowness of working speeds remains despite the use of equipment such as computers as Terry explained:

> *Visually impaired people, with the best computerised systems available, are at a disadvantage because of the amount of time and concentration it takes...Some people have got some great systems in operation but it's still unwieldy and time consuming and frustrating...you have to put in extra time, especially with the*

notes...I take time at the end of the day or lunch time, I nearly always work my lunch hour. It's got worse over the years, it's more difficult for sighted physios as well, but I've noticed that they have other strategies, like they can sit while they're having a cup of tea and they can be filling in notes and having a conversation at the same time. If you're visually impaired you need your equipment, you need to concentrate.

Hilary and Stephen, who are managers, estimate that they work at least an extra day each week to hold down their jobs:

I think it's something that shouldn't have to be done but in the real world I think it is unlikely that employers will give you that level of support, so if you want to survive in employment I think it's a question of accepting it and having to do it. The technology doesn't stop you from being slower as a visually impaired person. (Hilary)

I do about 46 hours purely to catch up with it all...I think a sighted person in this job would have to work more than 36 hours to do it but not as much as me. But then I'm glad I've got this job and to me it's worth putting the effort in. (Stephen)

Some of the physiotherapists felt obliged to work harder and longer in order to 'compensate' for their visual impairment. This could result in feelings of stress as Sarah explained:

The whole job is pressurised, you never go home at night forgetting about it, there's often a student report to do, or there's preparation to do for in-service training, or there's some notes to write up from a course you went on, or a course to attend at a weekend. There's always something and I just find that it takes over my whole life and I do nothing else but physio and of course things take longer because you can't see...I work considerably more hours, just to do a reasonable job. After a while that starts to wear a bit thin really.

Malcolm believes that '...there's no such thing as equal opportunities because it takes us longer'.

Josephine accepts the situation of having to work longer hours as being part of life as a disabled person:

You have to work harder and longer, oh yes. Because I'm part-time I can give the extra little bit and I don't mind really. That is life really...If you have a disability you have to run the extra mile.

Work overload and working long hours are widely recognised as important stressors at work (Hayward 1996, Porteous 1997). Mottram and Flin (1988) and Broom and Williams (1996) found that work overload is a common cause of stress among physiotherapists. Broom and Williams (1996) also highlight increased administration as a particular stressor for physiotherapists even though they have full access to print. In addition, the health professions are widely recognised as being high on the list of stressful occupations (Hayward 1996, Friend 1996, Broom and Williams 1996 Porteous 1997). The visually impaired physiotherapists are thus working in an environment that many non-disabled people find difficult.

Help from colleagues Thirteen of the 20 physiotherapists asked colleagues for some degree of help with administration. For three of the managers this posed no problem as they had access to secretarial assistance and were in a position to delegate. Stephen said:

> *You can delegate and make decisions. Although I create my own reports I don't have to spend any time making them look pretty I just give them to my secretary. If I have to do a presentation I can get the assistant to sort out the slides and make sure they look good, all I have to do is the talking and deal with the questions.*

Stephen also has a full-time physiotherapy assistant to help him with any task:

> *I've got a full-time assistant post entirely at my disposal which I negotiated...The Trust takes the view that physiotherapists are in short supply and they need to be facilitated in doing the job, be they visually impaired or not...I just put a business case forward for making me more effective in the job and the Trust could see it, there was no problem.*

Many of the physiotherapists asked physiotherapy assistants and other colleagues to help with reading notes and other administrative tasks. John said:

> *I'm lucky that the helpers, and all the staff generally, help with all the extra bits of paper that are around. The truth of the matter is that, as a blind person, you could get involved in form filling by putting it on the computer, but what the hell's the point because it's going to take an awful lot of time, and any skill and expertise I have is treating patients not inputting computer information.*

Some of the physiotherapists pointed out that the attitudes and behaviour of colleagues, particularly those in charge, were very important in reducing barriers created by administration. Josephine felt gratified that the head physiotherapist where she worked was so supportive:

> *I find that even though she is very high-powered, she's eager to get my ability to cope with the computer sorted out, the secretary to help me if necessary. I said I*

would pay for some extra secretarial help myself but she said 'No, no, we'll work it out another way'. She's very eager to keep me going which I find very flattering because there are youngsters about – but you see they definitely need us, there's a shortage.

Julia believes that the barrier posed by administration can become minor if the attitude of the person in charge is favourable:

Any superintendent worth anything will realise that the note-taking difficulties are minor compared with the advantages of employing us. When I was at B..., and I was working in out-patients, I could do 20 patients in an afternoon and it seemed quite natural that the secretary would fill all the cards in for me...it was a minor issue. The superintendent never raised it as a problem. It's down to your skills, how valued you make yourself and how reasonable your superintendent is.

These quotations illustrate the importance of supportive colleagues in coping with administration as well as other aspects of work. Support and congenial working relationships are widely recognised as factors which modify stress in the work place (Hayward 1996, Porteous 1997).

The Physical Environment

Barriers

Seventeen of the 20 physiotherapists mentioned that the physical environment could pose problems especially the environment of wards. This was a particular problem for totally blind people. John, who has worked in an outpatient setting for many years, said:

Nowadays, I must admit, my knees knock together with the idea of doing ward work again...Certainly when I talk to my year who I keep in contact with, all us 'totals' feel much the same...I didn't like the weekends because you had to go on to wards that you weren't familiar with, and you had to rely so much on your echo location for getting around. You can echo locate in familiar surroundings very quickly but when you go to unfamiliar ones you have to go a lot more slowly and, of course, you're that much more tense. The mental exhaustion of concentration in unfamiliar surroundings is quite tiresome.

Alice also works in an out-patient department but recalled her time on the wards:

Definitely it's easier to work in the out-patient department than struggle round the wards trying to find the patients...I haven't got enough sight to recognise a patient by any sort of facial feature unless I've seen them for a great many days. In most wards patients are moved around, as they become less acutely ill they're shunted up the ward...I'd go to the old bed first, and the patient had gone and then I'd have to start hunting for him so that was by far the worst thing. And I suppose the next difficult aspect was the anxiety about how many bottles, tubes and drips were likely to be attached to the patient. I would go very slowly and cautiously so as never to knock anything over, and luckily I never did, but that was an anxiety. And of course if the lighting wasn't very good then that added to all the problems.

Eric noticed an increasing number of barriers for visually impaired physiotherapists working on wards:

On the wards now the patients are more acutely ill, they're more disabled, the majority of patients on an orthopaedic ward need input now whereas say, even ten years ago, a lot of them would be independent. The patients now are often acutely ill, not just fractures, they've got drips and drains, vacuum pumps...it's a nightmare, I don't think a blind person can do that. Well I can do it with an assistant but we're much slower and the level of stress that I'm under is much, much higher...and just trying to find the patients is difficult because they move round.

Julia found the vases of flowers to be her major obstacle:

That's the thing I dreaded most, the vases of flowers on those wobbly little bedside tables. I think I probably felled about three in my ten years working in general hospitals. I was more worried about it than the drips and so on. The flowers seemed to make more mess than anything else if you did spill them.

Although the out-patient setting presented less problems, it was still mentioned by some physiotherapists as posing mobility barriers:

I have to be careful in my own department not to fall over wheelchairs, but you learn caution with age. When you've had a few bruised shins you get a bit more wary. (Julia)

I don't like the way we have a waiting room now, they all sit in the corridor, I find it difficult walking between rows of people with their legs out and I feel anxious lest I should kick one...So I tend to say jovially as I go in that direction 'How many legs, which side?!' but I don't enjoy it and I avoid going up there anymore than I have to. (Josephine)

Some of the physiotherapists had chosen to work in out-patient settings partly because of the difficulty of negotiating wards although this was rarely the only reason. Hilary said:

I definitely find it easier from the point of view of my visual impairment, there is no doubt about that. I think it is quite hard to work clinically in wards where everything's changing, but I don't think that was the only reason for my choice, I think I would have chosen out-patients anyway.

Malcolm's decision to work in an out-patient setting had also been influenced by his visual impairment:

I'm sure it had something to do with visual impairment. It was an interest but I think the fact also that one does not have to concern oneself quite so much with the mobility, the varying environment.

It was noted in chapter 5 that a high proportion of visually impaired physiotherapists work in out-patient settings.

Pam believes that finding and recognising patients on the wards is a particular problem for visually impaired physiotherapists with some sight:

I've worked with blind people in hospitals before and instantly people are calling to them 'I'm over here', 'This is Andy here' but I don't get any of that...when you're seem to be walking around OK they won't think 'She called me the wrong name because she didn't see me' that would never enter their heads.

This illustrates that even people with the same type of impairment can experience different barriers.

Some of the physiotherapists spoke of their need to concentrate very hard to cope with the environment, particularly the environment of wards. This was summed up by Alice:

With regard to the bottles and the bits and pieces, being very careful and thinking, using my brain to compensate for my eye sight. I really think that I've spent my whole life using my intelligence and every time there has been a deterioration then I've upped my concentration level and that is extremely exhausting.

Negotiating the physical environment is known to be difficult for visually impaired people (Bruce et al 1991, RNIB 1995, French and Swain 1997) and some other disabled people (French 1993b, Slack 1999). Some of the visually impaired employees interviewed by Simkiss et al (1998) highlighted the stress and the energy needed to cope with a hostile environment and how this could erode self-confidence and self-esteem. The needs of disabled people are rarely considered in health and safety policies, indeed disabled people are frequently regarded as a health and safety risk and excluded from premises on those grounds (Zarb 1995a). In 1999, however, a visually impaired physiotherapist was awarded compensation totalling £110,000 after tripping over a piece of hospital equipment and losing nearly all of her remaining sight (Physiotherapy Frontline 1999). Thus the law may be becoming more responsive to the needs of disabled people in the work place.

Some of the physiotherapists spoke of the barriers they experienced when working in intensive care units and the stress they felt under in that situation. One of the main problems was their inability to read the monitors. John explained:

> *One of the things that frightened me a little bit was an episode in intensive care, I was bagging a patient with a nurse, a very good nurse, I knew her quite well, and the consultant came over and said 'I hope that blood pressure machine isn't accurate' because the guy's blood pressure was about 250 over 160. Because I couldn't see it I was expecting this nurse to be aware of the machine but she was gaily bagging while I was doing the shaking and not paying attention to the instruments. I thought 'this is pretty risky' and it frightened me...When you're 'on-call' these days it's usually agency staff there and you have no idea of their reliability. So I thought it was potentially dangerous and I'd hate to think that just because I can't read a machine that somebody's life is in danger. I don't do intensive care work anymore.*

Eric found the equipment difficult too as well as the necessity to cover unfamiliar hospitals when doing 'on call' work:

> *I found it too difficult...there were so many hospitals we had to cover in the area, I wouldn't find the hospital never mind the ward, it was nonsense. Also it got much more high-tech especially in intensive care. You know, taking patients off ventilators, putting them back on. I didn't feel safe doing it. I was always uncertain but I did it when I was a junior, when I could see better, but I didn't enjoy it, in fact I hated it.*

Jenny and Lucy highlighted intensive care with babies as a particular problem. Jenny explained:

> *We have to treat quite a lot of babies here, tiny, tiny little kids, and that was really nerve wracking. I felt it was dangerous but I did it for a while.*

Some of the physiotherapists were, however, quite happy to work in intensive care units and did not find it particularly difficult or stressful especially as there were always a lot of nurses and other colleagues about. Hilary and Stephen found intensive care work easier than general ward work:

> *Well actually I found it easier because the nature of intensive care is that there are more staff so there was always someone available to ask. Most of the treatments that physiotherapists do in intensive care have to be done in a team so*

> there are usually two people treating…so things like the monitors didn't present a problem to me…I actually found intensive care quite a bit easier than general ward work. (Hilary)

> My first two years were spent most of the time on the wards including intensive care. The intensive care was the easiest bit which most people find very interesting. It was a smallish intensive care, only six beds, and I knew the staff extremely well and they knew me well…Now on normal wards you can't always find anybody. (Stephen)

This difference of opinion, regarding work in intensive care units, illustrates the way in which barriers are viewed dissimilarly by different individuals. Talking of occupational stress Porteous states:

> Environmental stressors affect individuals differently, people have varied coping strategies and individual reactions to stress. Coping is multi-dimensional and dependent on many situational factors and particularly the appraisal of the situation by the individual. (1997: 229)

Strategies

Help from colleagues A major strategy used by the physiotherapists working on wards was asking help of their colleagues. Finding someone to ask for help was not, however, always straightforward as Malcolm pointed out:

> I always asked at the desk beforehand. In fact that became more difficult because more often than not there was no one at the desk, fewer staff you see, so not being able to look at the cardex I couldn't get to know where people were.

Some of the physiotherapists believed that the ward staff had to be 'won over' and educated before they would give the help required. Hilary explained:

> I think probably forming good relationships with the ward staff was important. Making sure that they understand your needs, that you do have a visual impairment and that there is a small amount of assistance that you will require.

Stephen also mentioned the need to form good relationships with ward staff to ensure sufficient assistance:

> Personality is one thing and also you need to know what you're talking about. Personality and a good knowledge of physiotherapy and the gift of the gab. Those are the three important things.

These quotations illustrate how the physiotherapists had to take the initiative and develop skills to 'manage' their working relationships. Kitchen et al (1998), in their study of disabled people, point out the poor attitudes of employers and their ignorance of disability, and Morris (1991) talks of the delicate and problematic nature of relationships between disabled and non-disabled people and how disabled people are forced to take the initiative and the responsibility for managing relationships.

A major strategy used by those physiotherapists who disliked intensive care work was avoidance. This was often achieved through negotiation with colleagues which became easier as the physiotherapists became more senior. Malcolm said:

> *I decided it was wiser to avoid it. They did ask me to submit a written account of reasons which I did and there was no hassle at all about it...There was one incident where a patient needed suction and there were just no staff to do it and I felt that my whole treatment of that patient was inadequate. I wasn't getting the staff back-up that I had in the past because there were less staff. About three years before I gave it up I was thinking 'Hey, should I be doing this?'.*

For some of the physiotherapists negotiation has been precarious and dependent upon the goodwill of a particular person:

> *I don't have to do it, but they have said that if they get very desperate they will teach me and I will have to do it but I hope that never arises...I made it perfectly clear to them that I'd never done intensive care work and they said 'That's OK but if we really hit a crisis then we might have to teach you and we'll give you the full back-up of teaching you before we expect you to do it'. ...I don't know whether we can, as such, say we want to be exempt from it. I think, according to your contract, you are expected to do weekend and 'on-call' work...I don't know what their intentions are really but I think if it ever came to it I would have to say 'Look, I don't feel competent to do it' and hopefully, now that I'm in post, I couldn't be kicked out.* (Sarah)

> *I've avoided it (intensive care) as a placement, thank God, but I had to do it as 'on-call' and weekends in my previous job at N... but it was a small hospital and I felt that I just about coped with it. My present hospital is very large with a large ICU (intensive care unit) and you have to supervise juniors so I had a long talk to the superintendent and was exempted from doing on-calls and weekends...She was a very good superintendent, she's gone now, you can't rely on the same response from someone else.* (Sharron)

Sheila and Julia were not expected to cope with intensive care work on their own, a situation that was decided for them by their managers:

Employment: Barriers and Coping Strategies 135

> *At U... I did do 'on-calls' and I found it quite hard because it was my first job and I had to do night work in strange places. But I coped and I found that the nursing staff were helpful but it was quite a strain and a stress. But whenever you talked to her (the superintendent) there was never any feeling that she didn't think that you could do things. In my next job I did get the impression that the superintendent...well she took me on but there was that feeling that I couldn't possibly do the same job that she could do with sight. I found that with the weekend work I was quite relieved to find that she didn't want me to do Sundays on my own. I didn't make a fuss about it because I was rather pleased...It was one occasion when her attitude was quite a perk.* (Julia)

> *In S... where intensive care was more specialised, I had a physiotherapist working with me on a weekend. I think that was something that the superintendent organised for me, I didn't ask for it...They never made any big thing about it...I'm afraid I just accepted it and was grateful.* (Sheila)

Pam demanded that she be taken off the 'on-call' rota and felt that her senior position helped as it is cheaper to employ junior staff during unsocial hours.

Colleagues were very important to the visually impaired physiotherapists in overcoming or minimising various environmental barriers. Some of the help was highly formalised, for example the use of secretarial time, but mostly it was haphazard, unreliable and dependent on how well the physiotherapists were able to form co-operative relationships. Situations and events which are unpredictable and where the individual feels he or she has little control have the potential to be very stressful (Atkinson et al 1993). Lack of control at work is also associated with poor self-esteem and low job satisfaction (Hayward 1996). Lack of control was more likely among those physiotherapists who were in clinical grades and, therefore, lacked power within the organisation. This indicates how barriers can be easier to remove when disabled individuals have senior positions. Similar findings were reported in Chapter 3, regarding disabled health and welfare professionals, and it was noted in chapter 1 that the norms and ideologies of institutions and organisations are maintained by powerful groups.

Help from patients and clients Most of the physiotherapists spoke highly of the help they received from patients and clients. Julia explained:

> *Well I didn't need to ask for help in the wards I worked on every day because once the patients knew who you were they couldn't wait to shout 'Stop there's a table!'. You'd say 'Where's Mr. Brown?' and they'd say 'Hang on, I'll go and look for him'. The patients were my first ally.*

Malcolm had similar experiences:

> *They would assist you in locating them themselves by shouting out "Ere I am' and they would ensure that you didn't clobber into something on your way out of the ward by instructing you verbally or, if they were fit enough, actually escorting you out. I've always found the patients very helpful if they were well enough to be so...I've had the odd patient who has asked me 'Are you going to be able to do it all right?' and I say 'Yes, there's no problem, but if you feel unhappy about anything please say'. But that's very rare...When you think they have never come across one (a blind person) they really take it very well.*

As Pam noted, physiotherapists with some sight tend not to get this kind of assistance, either from colleagues or from patients and clients, because people do not know or understand the extent of their visual impairment. This shows that visual impairment (as opposed to total blindness) can give rise to ambiguity and lack of understanding which, in turn, can lead to different kinds of barriers (French 1997c).

Some of the physiotherapists voiced surprise that patients and clients were not more concerned about visual impairment. Andrea said:

> *They're very good, very accepting, not worried at all about having a totally blind physio work with them. One or two queries about whether I'd be able to manage this or that, but literally only two or three over the whole of the years I've been working which is not bad going. They've been very friendly and very chatty and obviously quite interested as well.*

In a survey of disabled physiotherapists (CSP 1996) only 3.5 per cent had found that patients and clients were reluctant to be treated by them.

Some of the physiotherapists speculated on why patients and clients had so much confidence in them. Josephine felt that some of them did not notice her total blindness:

> *In an out-patient setting they come into the cubicle that I'm using and I know where everything is in that cubicle and so they don't know until they've handed me their trust that I can't see at all. They imagine that I have some partial sight...When they do notice they already trust you. There must be some who think 'Gosh, is she safe with that electrical apparatus?' but I've never had anybody decline!*

Hilary and Julia agree but also think that patients and clients have idealised and mystical ideas about blindness which gives them confidence in the blind physiotherapist. Hilary said:

> *There is also this feeling that people have that someone with a visual impairment has this wonderful sixth sense that has got something to do with the 'healing hand'. I think it's entirely mythical. I think it's because we use the other four senses a lot more and people find that quite strange to observe.*

Stephen is prepared to use the idealised views of his patients and clients to his advantage although he is aware of the ethical dilemma it poses:

Most people think you do better than others because you are blind, which is crazy to be honest, but use it to your advantage I say, why not? There are so many disadvantages. If a patient believes in you you're half way there really, perhaps I shouldn't say this...but you could almost be unqualified and get away with it. This puts a great responsibility on you because if people put a lot of trust in you you shouldn't be dishonest.

Disabled people, including those with visual impairments, are frequently stereotyped as helpless and dependent (Barnes 1992, French and Swain 1997). Some of the physiotherapists noted that they are treated far more positively by patients and clients than by the public as a whole. Their professional role appears to be effective in conferring perceptions of competence, rather than inadequacy, upon them.

Meetings

Barriers

The majority of the physiotherapists did not need to attend many meetings but seven did speak of the barriers they presented. The main problems they experienced were the inability to see non-verbal communication and to read papers which were not circulated in advance. This is illustrated in the following quotations:

I've worked in some very difficult situations with some very autocratic doctors and at team meetings it's a problem of picking up their non-verbal communication, when they're getting angry and things. To a certain extent it affected my ability to handle difficult situations, you know, knowing when it might be best to say nothing. (Sharron)

Yes, they do pass papers around...and yes you do miss out sometimes...And people won't make excuses for you that you couldn't read the information, they just think you're being inadequate and not fulfilling your role even if they haven't given you material in an accessible format. I also find a problem, and I find this socially as well, in that I'm not very good at interacting, I've got better at it, in meetings particularly, but because you can't make eye contact with somebody I find it difficult to get into a conversation. But I get enough about feeling and mood from their voices, silences and so on. (Sarah)

Talking of meetings Robert concluded that 'There's no determination to be unhelpful but people are not very perceptive either'.

There is a large psychological literature on the importance of non-verbal communication in personal interaction. Much of non-verbal communication is visual although emotion is also expressed through non-verbal vocalisations (Argyle 1988).

Strategies

The strategies the physiotherapists mentioned were mostly in terms of being open and assertive. Hilary asks for papers to be provided in advance and tells people that she is unable to respond to non-verbal communication. Stephen makes it clear that if documents are not made accessible to him he will not be responsible for the decisions that are made, though he wonders how much other people are able to assimilate the information:

> *Most of the time I'm belligerent and say 'Sorry I'm not party to this decision because I haven't had an opportunity to read the paper and I want that minuted'. But, to be honest, if it's a 40 page document nobody else has read it well enough to make sensible decisions.*

Hilary tries to resolve the situation in advance:

> *One of the things that I do find difficult is when people bring documents to a meeting for consideration and they haven't circulated them beforehand. That is difficult because other people will sit there and scan it and I'm unable to do that. So what I try to do is...make sure that other members of the group are aware and that they try to get documents to me beforehand. That works to a certain extent but inevitably it doesn't always work.*

Stephen relies on the force of his personality to overcome his lack of non-verbal information in meetings:

> *I think I use other characteristics to my advantage. Humour is a very powerful one, being witty is a great asset...being an introvert is no good if you're a visually impaired physio, the two things don't go together, you have a real battle on your hands then because how else can you communicate that bit of warmth? Perhaps humour is not quite the right word, somehow you need to bring somebody's personality out without being able to see them, for that you need wit and intuition I suppose. You need to be a good communicator.*

Hilary finds that if she is chairing a meeting she has the power to minimise the barriers both in terms of communication and information:

> *I think it nearly always comes down to the politics of dealing with the situation, you miss the glance between people, of agreement or dissent, or you miss that someone is agitated by a statement that you've just made or doesn't under-*

stand a statement that you've just made, or is disagreeing or feeling unhappy, or threatened...The way that I deal with that, if I'm chairing a group, is that I go round to every individual and say 'Is that OK with you?'...If I'm a member of the group, and not chairing it, it isn't in my power to do that...and usually if I'm chairing it I'm in possession of most of the information before I get there.

Health and welfare professionals with sensory impairments also found that chairing meetings gave them more control in terms of communication and information, as discussed in chapter 3.

Behaviour of Colleagues as a Barrier and as a Coping Strategy

Seeking the help of colleagues has been highlighted as a coping strategy, with regard to particular barriers, throughout this chapter and chapter 3 which considered disabled health and welfare professionals. Most of the physiotherapists spoke highly of the assistance they were given by colleagues as well as their favourable attitudes and behaviour towards them as disabled people. Eric, for example, found his manager helped him to re-negotiate his job when he found it was becoming too difficult:

I think that the stress just became so great, it was my fear of litigation...So I went to my immediate boss and said 'I can't do it anymore'. I told her about the counselling and she said 'Well, we can try and get you a half and half post...so you can just do the arthritis patients, which I know you find interesting and are very experienced with, and some counselling'.

John was very positive about the way he was treated by colleagues:

I've been very lucky, yes...There have been a large number of staff through here and I've not had any clashes of personality or any snipes or anything about the fact that I don't do the full amount of paper work. They've all been brilliant.

Some of the physiotherapists did, however, find the help they received from colleagues variable and haphazard. Sheila said:

I always put the patient first so if something needed to happen for the good of that patient I would feel it my responsibility to make sure it happened, therefore if I couldn't do it for them I'd need to ask a nurse's help. There were some really helpful nurses and some that weren't.

Simkiss et al (1998) found, from the interviews they conducted with visually impaired employees, that the help they received varied greatly with individuals despite the policy of the work place. This was also the experience of many of the health and welfare professionals discussed in chapter 3.

Most of the physiotherapists could recall isolated instances when colleagues had had poor attitudes towards them which served as barriers:

I think I've been lucky, I think I've had a good career. I have met the occasional person who has not liked the fact that I can't see very well, but most of the people I've worked with have been very supportive, and that's including the medical profession...I did apply for a job at N... and didn't get it. They seemed to be worried that I'd fall over everything! That was way back in the early seventies. (Lucy)

In the main people were helpful. I had one unpleasant experience with a registrar, when I was on-call, who felt that it was inappropriate for visually impaired people to work in health care. I made sure I told him what sort of people I felt were inappropriate! That was settled between me and him...But on the whole I've found that people are very helpful. (Hilary)

Some of the physiotherapists with some sight had experienced negative attitudes and lack of understanding from colleagues who failed to appreciate or believe the extent of their visual impairment. Pam said:

I'm a registered blind person but they haven't got a clue...If I stay in one building I'm fine, it's only when I go over to G...that I get really lost...and one of the physios says, 'So you're not talking to me today!' because I've walked right past them...and I've worked with them for years; oh dear!...I just say 'I didn't see you' but they don't seem to learn.

This kind of treatment, which was also noted by a visually impaired social worker in chapter 3, can be regarded as bullying behaviour and harassment. In a survey of disabled physiotherapists (CSP 1996), 17.7 per cent reported discrimination and harassment from other physiotherapists, 24.4 per cent from managers and 8.9 per cent from other health care workers. Similarly, the disabled physiotherapists in the Disability Network (a pressure group of disabled physiotherapists) of the CSP reported lack of respect and awareness, teasing and a lack of regard for their views by non-disabled colleagues (Physiotherapy Frontline 1997b).

Minimisation, Compensation and Openness

As noted in chapter 6, Barnes (1996) highlights three major strategies which he has used at various stages of his life to cope as a visually impaired person; minimisation, compensation and openness. Similar strategies were also described by Goffman (1968). All of these strategies were used by the visually impaired physiotherapists.

Minimisation refers to attempts by disabled people to play down their impairments and disabilities in order to appear 'normal' and therefore to be acceptable. Sarah said:

I try to cover it up (disability) as much as possible. I ask to work in the same cubicle so that I'm not stumbling over things all the time...so that I can appear to be much more sighted in front of people and much more confident. I try to put on as normal a front as possible...and that's a tremendous strain. Walking round the department trying to look sighted is very stressful.

Simkiss et al (1998), in their study of visually impaired employees, found that some people disguised disability as a way of reducing discrimination. One research respondent said 'I disguise it as much as possible...whether you like it or not you're regarded as a second-class citizen' (1998: 102).

Sharron traced the strategy of minimisation back to childhood experiences:

I think a lot of it comes from me, the feeling that I ought to be able to cope...I want to appear to cope so I avoid asking or letting people know that I have a problem. It creates a huge anxiety for me...It's been a problem for me right from school days. I did have some bad experiences at school where teachers just didn't believe that I couldn't see...I was teased and bullied at school and I think that did affect my ability to deal with my eye sight problem really. I think it's difficult because my eye sight is of a level where, for most things, you do cope but it's more of an anxiety thing about whether you are going to cope and not knowing until you are in that situation.

Barnes defines compensation as 'The development of socially valued attributes which deflect attention from subjective limitations' (1996: 40). Compensation often involves the disabled person in attempts to work harder or to achieve more than non-disabled people. The tendency of disabled people to compensate was noted by Kitchen et al (1998) in their study of disabled people at work.

A few of the physiotherapists did talk about their need to prove themselves to others and to compensate for their visual limitations. Alice traced this back to childhood experiences:

Even at 18, I was very conscious that I needed to place myself in the world as somebody who could still be significant even though I was disabled. I put a huge amount of effort into things because I did not want to be written off as an inadequate person...I'm always trying to prove myself. I think that says something about my parents...They both found that my being visually impaired was a desperately sad situation for them and therefore I wanted to prove myself, I wanted to buy their approval...and when people used to ask me as a student 'Why are you working so hard?' I would actually say 'Because I want to please my parents'...It has taken a lot of effort for me to learn to ask for help and admit my blindness, but now I do and it's OK. It's all to do with trying to compensate, it's very exhausting.

Similarly, McDonald (1996), who is physically disabled, says that his family always encouraged him to work twice as hard as everybody else to compensate for his disability and his minority ethnic status.

The effects of childhood experiences on the coping strategies used by disabled people is an area which needs investigation. Several of the visually impaired physiotherapists spoke of the adverse effects that various childhood experiences, for example attending special school, attending mainstream school and the behaviour of parents, had had on them as adults.

Malcolm and Sarah also spoke about compensation as one of their coping strategies:

...compensation, I've tried that, to my cost probably. You know, having perfect notes, getting through more patients than other people...If you try to do it when you're older you just can't manage to do it at the same rate, you can survive it better when you're younger. (Malcolm)

I've worked full time for 22 years and I've never had any time off apart from a few weeks to train for the dog...well I've had eight days in 22 years. My sick record is super but, you know, it's partly because you never want to give people cause to say 'Oh dear, we've got problems with her in more ways than one'. So I do tend to push myself...I'm determined that nobody will ever say 'You're not doing that adequately'. (Sarah)

Minimisation of disability and compensation tend to be damaging strategies but they should not be regarded as irrational. Disabled people are not always well accepted and they do face hostile attitudes and discrimination which encourage these strategies. As one of the members of the Disability Network said:

Physiotherapy has an image of being whole and complete, and the acknowledgement that there is a physiotherapist with a physical disability jars with that image. (Physiotherapy Frontline 1995: 18)

Most of the physiotherapists used openness about their visual impairments, where they made their needs known, as a major coping strategy:

I do tell people, I tell anybody, even if somebody comes for an informal visit and I'm showing them the hospital I tell them because I find it so much easier. You can be caught out if you don't and you can look stupid...Sometimes people say 'Have you forgotten your glasses today?' and I find it simpler to say 'Well actually I'm registered blind and I use a white stick to walk about outside'. I put it as bluntly as that. (Charlotte)

I would be quite open about the fact that I was visually impaired or registered blind and that this is the way I cope with things...they can take it or leave it...I don't think its a question of harping on about your own needs or anything like that but not being afraid to say 'Yes, that's the situation and I need this, that or the other'. (Robert)

Some of the physiotherapists had become more open about their visual impairments as their sight had deteriorated. Others had become more open as they had grown older. This is also likely to be related to their more senior positions at work where greater power makes openness less of a risk:

I tend to ask more and defend myself a bit more than I used to. I'm more open than I used to be. Older and more experienced is probably the reason. You tend to say 'Hey look, can this be adapted, can this be adjusted?'...Before I might have 'put up' and 'shut up'. (Malcolm)

I've learned over the years to be very much more open and extrovert. In learning disabilities I always know what I can do and what I can't do and if I want someone to throw a ball to the client and catch it again – well there's no way I'm going to try and do it. (Julia)

Conclusion

This account illustrates that the visually impaired physiotherapists experienced institutional discrimination in their employment. They experienced barriers at all three levels of the SEAwall of institutional discrimination (Swain et al 1998) which was discussed in chapter 1. At the structural level the norms and ideologies of hospitals, and other health care establishments, are geared towards non-disabled people, for example the assumption that employees can read print and can drive. The physiotherapists also experienced many environmental barriers, for example the haphazard environment of wards and the lack of accessible equipment. Many examples of attitudinal barriers were also voiced.

These barriers are similar to those highlighted in the first phase of the study (see chapter 5) Attitudinal discrimination appear to have reduced perhaps aided by the Disability Discrimination Act (1995), other government initiatives (for example Access to Work) and equal opportunity policies. On the other hand, changes in health care practice, especially since the NHS and Community Care Act, have made work more difficult for some of the physiotherapists due, for example, to the rapid turnover of patients, the increase in community rather than hospital based practice and the fact that a high proportion of hospital patients are seriously ill. The physiotherapists also experienced barriers from within themselves, such as feelings of inadequacy and fear. These barriers do not fit so readily into the framework of the social model of disability or institutional discrimination although they do, in part, result from the disabling environment.

The strategies the physiotherapists used to overcome, minimise or manage these barriers included the avoidance of difficult situations, taking advantage of the Access to Work scheme, seeking help from colleagues, patients and clients, adapting medical equipment and taking more time. Cognitive strategies, such as increased concentration, an enhanced memory and the use of echo location, were also employed but were regarded as stressful and exhausting when used in isolation. Most of the physiotherapists were open about their needs although some attempted to minimise the problems they encountered or to over-compensate for them.

The strategies the physiotherapists adopted depended, not only on their own personal style and background, but on government policy, their seniority within the organisation, their age, the attitudes and behaviour of their employers and colleagues, the particular situations they were in and the type of organisations in which they were employed. Most of the physiotherapists were eager to remove the barriers they experienced by changing the environment rather than attempting to change themselves.

Chapter 8

The Changing Work Environment: Its Impact on Visually Impaired Physiotherapists

During the period between the first and second phases of this study, considerable changes occurred within the NHS, within disability legislation and politics and (arguably) within the attitudes and behaviour of society towards disabled people. This chapter will draw on the 20 interviews in the second phase of the study to illustrate the ways in which these changes have impacted upon the working lives of visually impaired physiotherapists. It will also examine the reflections of the physiotherapists on their promotion within the physiotherapy profession, their job satisfaction and their attitudes towards physiotherapy as a suitable career for visually impaired people in the future.

The Impact of The NHS and Community Care Act (1990) on the Working Lives of Visually Impaired Physiotherapists

The NHS and Community Care Act (1990) is wide-ranging legislation which introduced ideas of the market into health and community care. The impact of this on the visually impaired physiotherapists is mainly an increase in administrative work, a greater proportion of physiotherapy taking place in the community and an increased speed of work. Two of the visually impaired physiotherapists, who are managers, noted how their entire job had changed. Charlotte said:

> *I don't think that in the old days, when I started, that you had the sort of manager that I am now. You had clinical managers…I don't think anybody spent time on, well like an annual report that I've just done, a business plan will come up in the Autumn, I've done a paper recently on risk management, I've done a paper on coping with students without any funding coming in, I have a meeting with purchasing agencies and we discuss new projects and how we are going to get funding, putting in bids for money from the Department of Health. I don't think those sort of things went on before.*

Some of the physiotherapists spoke of the increase in administration since the NHS reforms. Sharron said:

> *There's a lot more paper work. I can read print but I'm slow and I find the statistics a real chore...People are a lot busier and that has affected people's willingness and ability to help. I think you are expected to get on with it, there is so much emphasis on efficiency and effectiveness.*

Other physiotherapists spoke of increased job insecurity and increased pressure to work faster and with less resources. Andrea said:

> *You're always under pressure now to do that little bit extra and sometimes you feel that you haven't got enough time for patient care...Trusts are always talking about how they need to cut back, they always seem to be in debt, they threaten redundancies and you think 'Who will it be next?'. You try to convince yourself that you are needed where you are. And would they dare to get rid of a disabled person?*

Job insecurity is highlighted by Hayward (1996) as a common cause of stress at work.

Despite equal opportunity policies, the Disability Discrimination Act (1995) and less blatant discrimination against visually impaired physiotherapists, the changing environment of health care, which is connected to some extent with the NHS and Community Care Act, has made some aspects of the job more difficult for visually impaired physiotherapists. Similar barriers were emphasised in phase one of the study (see chapter 5) though they may have become more intense. Fifty per cent of the visually impaired physiotherapists in phase one of the study reported that the job had become more difficult because of increased administration and an increase in community practice. Thirteen per cent, however, found the job easier mainly because of improved attitudes towards disabled people.

Promotion

Some of the physiotherapists were inhibited about applying for promotion because of the barriers they believed they would experience. Julia said:

> *To be a service head means an awful lot of reading, an awful lot of travelling between sites, an awful lot of going to meetings, relating to people and I think that we are at a disadvantage because we can't move freely around, we can't recognise people, we can't read on the spot and react to little messages passed or whatever. I know there are two blind service heads but I don't know how they do their jobs basically.*

Stephen, who is a district manager, is not sure why he has not progressed even higher up the scale but he feels that the barriers he would face as a blind person is probably a factor:

> *It's funny because my brother is one of these high-flying guys, he's doing very well...He said to me a few months ago...'Isn't it about time you moved up?' and I had to say to him that I think I could cope with it if I could see, I would like to have gone into a consultancy type thing in physiotherapy...or gone into health management, but I don't know whether I could have coped with it...But then David Blunkett does it, so I don't know.*

Sharron is apprehensive about new employment and relates this, in part, to visual impairment:

> *I think it's very difficult to be objective about whether you have been discriminated against, it's very difficult to tell. Applying for jobs is quite an anxious time for me, there are all the fears of 'How will I cope with this, how will I cope with that?'.*

Charlotte also pointed out the difficulty of knowing whether or not discrimination is taking place especially as an older woman:

> *I applied for two jobs before Christmas...I thought 'If I'm going to move, it's now or never'. I didn't get an interview for either of them but it's very difficult to say why I didn't because I feel; I'm a woman, I'm over 50 now and I'm visually impaired. With one of the jobs I knew very definitely that driving would be of use but they said, in very big print 'WE ARE AN EQUAL OPPORTUNITIES EMPLOYER' and it didn't actually say that driving was an essential part...You can't tell, can you, why you don't get posts.*

Ben feels that his visual impairment may have hindered his promotion within physiotherapy education although he too is unsure:

> *I've been a senior lecturer now ever since 1978 and that is a long time to be a senior lecturer...I've applied for Principal jobs in the past and never got one and I think it's partly due to the visual thing, there may be other aspects as well, I don't know.*

Similar doubts were expressed by disabled people interviewed by Duckett (2000).

Some of the physiotherapists had experienced attitudinal barriers when applying for jobs. Pam recalled:

> *We were chatting for half an hour all nice and then I told her where I trained and she completely changed and didn't even offer me an application form. I was going to ask her but I thought 'No, you'll be fighting the whole way, it's just not*

worth it'...I'm not confrontational...if you're struggling, especially in the first few weeks to find your way around, you don't want someone saying 'I told you you couldn't do this job'.

Some of the visually impaired employees interviewed by Simkiss et al (1998) had similar experiences. One respondent said:

They don't call it discrimination, they just tell you they're not interested – you don't know whether they're discriminating or not...the problem is if you proved discrimination you wouldn't want to work there anyway. (1998: 103)

Similar points were made by disabled people interviewed by Duckett (2000) where the interview was viewed as a place where discrimination could be practised covertly.

Robert, who is a district manager, experienced gender discrimination earlier in his career:

I remember writing off to N... for a vacancy. I said 'I'm a blind physio and a male physio' and I got this letter back (this is the early 70s) saying 'We have no facilities for males!'. They used the male thing on that one. On the visual aspect there has never been anything explicit but you feel you've got to work that much harder at it to obtain the posts you want to get over the years.

Some of the visually impaired physiotherapists connected their lack of promotion with factors other than visual impairment. Sandra said:

The jobs that I've gone for I've tended to get. I think they've been jobs that other people might not want. I haven't liked jobs in big hospitals, I always try to avoid that sort of situation...I don't think it's from a visual point of view really...I don't like acute physiotherapy very much, I find it easier to do more chronic things. I just prefer small places.

Like many women Alice always saw work as secondary to her family responsibilities:

I'm a qualified teacher and I'm a senior 1. I didn't want to go any higher. I avoided it because I got married and I didn't want a full-time job. I decided that being married and having children was my priority and the work would be second to that and be part-time...I only did teaching because I was sort of persuaded to do it...It wasn't my choice at all. I didn't teach for long.

In a survey of disabled physiotherapists (CSP 1996), 24.4 per cent of respondents believed they had been discriminated against in terms of promotion. Promotion prospects were also cited as a problem by the disabled physiotherapists in the Disability Network of the CSP. The belief that visual impairment had had an adverse effect on promotion was evident among the visually impaired physiotherapists in the first phase of the study where 37 per cent agreed that it had had an adverse effect and 62 per cent had avoided promotion because of visual impairment. It is not possible to say from these data whether promotion prospects for visually impaired physiotherapists has changed.

Job Satisfaction

Job satisfaction is a multi-faceted concept and has been defined by Porteous as 'a set of feelings about work' (1997: 36). Despite the barriers the physiotherapists experienced in their working lives most reported high job satisfaction. Lucy, who is soon to retire, said:

> *It's been a very satisfying job...I think I've had a very worthwhile and satisfying career...It's given me a good life, an opportunity to travel, to meet all sorts of people and to have a very fulfilled life because, OK physio has its limitations, but I think I've done something useful for a few people over the years, I think I've contributed.*

Josephine's major satisfaction in her work as a physiotherapist has come from being able to give to other people rather than always being the recipient of help:

> *I feel that it's one of the few jobs where you are giving to others. I know it sounds horribly saintly, but you don't want to always be helped, or receiving...to be helpful as a blind person is not always easy.*

Alice is satisfied with her work as a physiotherapist both in terms of being a disabled person and in terms of being a woman:

> *I'm really glad I trained as a physio. I think it's one of the best careers for a woman...you can do it at almost any level, as much or as little as you like, you can be married, you can have children, you can get back to it, you can almost pick your hours. It's given me a valid role as a disabled person which I feel is very important because it's very easy to feel inadequate and inferior. To be professionally qualified is a great morale booster, definitely. I always feel proud to say that I'm a physiotherapist.*

These quotations suggest that having a professional career counteracts some of the negative attitudes people have about visual impairment. Similar views were expressed by some of the private practitioners in the first phase of the study who felt that they had a valuable role within their communities and one which helped to integrate them as blind people.

For many of the physiotherapists their job satisfaction had risen despite increasing barriers. Julia, who works as a manager with clients with learning difficulties, has been involved in the move from institutional to community living and now works within the community. She said:

> *I think in a way it (job satisfaction) has gone up...It's very stimulating because you come into contact with a lot of different people. Since we came out of L... (the institution) we've had referrals from people who have never had treatment before who live with their families, so we've met an awful lot more families and carers and I find that keeping all the balls going in the air at once is really stimulating.*

John explains his increase in job satisfaction in terms of his increased expertise:

> *I think it has got better because as you get more expertise there are more things you can handle, more things that you recognise, and therefore you probably have a better success rate. That's what gives me the most pleasure – when a patient comes in and says 'I'm so much better'...That to me has always been my biggest pleasure in work.*

Sheila believes that her job satisfaction has risen because she is now in a position to specialise.

For some of the physiotherapists, however, their job satisfaction had gone down. Robert and Hilary, who are managers, related this to the restructuring of the NHS and the increased pressures that have ensued. Robert said:

> *I would say it has gone down, but that is largely to do with the NHS, the structure and organisation, not to do with visual impairment aspects of life...People are fed up with the organisation, with the politics of it, the bureaucracy, the increase in paper work, the contracts, all this stuff.*

Ben finds working in large universities less satisfying that small NHS physiotherapy colleges where he used to work:

> *I must say that I'm not a lover of large scale things, I'm not a lover of vast organisations and doing things in big ways. In terms of relationships with students I got more satisfaction in days gone by in smaller colleges where I knew the students better. I'm removed from the students here and I think it's because there are so many of them...and I can't work out who the hell is who most of the time...In terms of the actual job, yes, I was a bit happier with the smaller groups...if you get a practical group by yourself it is quite a lot, 22, 24. That does happen sometimes, particularly in anatomy, that becomes a bit of a struggle.*

Sarah, Sharron and Sandra have always felt relatively dissatisfied with physiotherapy. Sarah, who has been a senior physiotherapist for 20 years, feels inadequate and relates this to feelings about herself as a visually impaired person as well as lack of support:

> *I don't think I feel totally fulfilled in my job but that's because of lots of different things...I do have an inferiority complex...I always feel that people know much more than me and I think that comes from the fact that I can't see. As a small child I wasn't like that and it was when I went away to a blind school that I lost my confidence...This inferiority complex is compounded by the fact that I often feel that I'm working at half measures, that because of my sight problem I'm cutting corners because I haven't got the where-with-all to do things properly...I haven't wanted to take on extra responsibilities and maybe I haven't been quite so fulfilled because of that...I've never explored new territory because I don't feel adequate and supported to do it.*

Sharron feels that physiotherapy was not her choice. She also feels an outsider in physiotherapy in terms of social class:

> *I've always been relatively dissatisfied. Physiotherapy was not my choice really, it was something I was advised to do...I don't come from a family where education is valued...but people thought it was important for me to be educated and I did get three 'A' levels. Class was another factor in feeling unable to cope, I came from a working class background and wasn't used to the middle-class way of doing things.*

It was noted in chapter 5 that many more visually impaired physiotherapists, than sighted physiotherapists, come from non-professional backgrounds.

Sandra has never enjoyed her work as a physiotherapist and feels that she would not be in the profession if she were not visually impaired:

> *I just don't like the job, it's got nothing to do with visual impairment. Well, indirectly, it has because I don't think I would have done it if I hadn't been visually impaired.*

The overall high job satisfaction of visually impaired physiotherapists reflects the findings in the first phase of the study (see chapter 5) where 77 per cent of the visually impaired physiotherapists were either satisfied or very satisfied with their work. It also supports the findings of Simkiss et al (1998) who found that 69 per cent of the visually impaired professional workers they interviewed were satisfied. In general studies of job satisfaction, professional workers are, on balance, more satisfied than non-professional workers (Porteous 1997). It is not possible to conclude from these data whether or not the job satisfaction of visually impaired physiotherapists has changed.

The Suitability of Physiotherapy as a Career for Visually Impaired People

Most of the physiotherapists felt that, despite the barriers, physiotherapy was still a suitable career for visually impaired people. Lucy said:

> *If you have a bent to do anything towards the medical or caring professions, physiotherapy is by far the most suitable and I think that the degree qualification gives you a much wider scope than we had...I think we still need pressure groups to make sure it still happens, that's why I'm so keen on the ABCP.*

Pam and Charlotte are undaunted by the growing technical and academic nature of physiotherapy believing it is still essentially a 'hands-on' and 'people' profession:

> *It doesn't have to be technical at all. We're going back into muscles now and 'hands-on' – it's swings and roundabouts.* (Pam)

> *I think they have become too academic...it's still a people profession, one-to-one, communicating.* (Charlotte)

Some of the physiotherapists, particularly those who are totally blind, thought the profession was suitable for people with some sight but were doubtful that totally blind people could still manage every aspect of the work:

> *I think it's going to be very difficult for a totally blind physiotherapist to compete and have the same job opportunities as a sighted physiotherapist...I'm thinking of intensive care work, some of the machinery. The better the eye sight the more you can participate. Even big class work is really out for blind physios. The increase in community work is another problem. There are many things that negate against us so we have to offer something exceptional to compensate for that...Though there are big parts of physio that involve exercise, massage and manipulations, where I actually think we've got the edge over sighted people because we do use our sense of touch to perfection. At the same time there's a lot more apparatus, there's a lot more note taking, a lot more reading that must be done, there are many deficits that we experience.* (Josephine)

> *It's probably a case of choosing the right sort of niche once you've qualified. It's difficult because there has always been this philosophy that we can do everything and I've never gone along with that. I think it's a bit crazy sending us into ICU (intensive care units). That sort of thing does need acknowledging. It's difficult because you don't want to give people a different qualification but I think maybe it should be accepted that there might be certain areas that we can't do.* (Sharron)

Robert believes that there is still much that visually impaired people can achieve within physiotherapy provided the support is available:

> *I think it has become more difficult...but there are certainly skills that they could home in on where they could do a very satisfactory job for a working life. But things have changed, there's a lot more health education, health promotion, presentational aspects of the work, record keeping is much more wide ranging, so there would need to be some good support mechanisms in place.*

Stephen believes that the attitude of the CSP is crucial with regard to the survival of visually impaired people in the profession and, like Sharron, brings up the issue of whether visually impaired people need to be able to do every aspect of the job:

> *It's the whole ethos of whether the Chartered Society wants blind physiotherapists in their midst...Then you get into an argument about the nature of physiotherapy. Should you be able to cope with all fields of physiotherapy or is it good enough to do some parts of physiotherapy? Now I think that blind and partially sighted people can do most of physiotherapy. There are very few generic physios around these days anyway.*

Most of the physiotherapists felt that the attitudes of their professional body towards visually impaired physiotherapists, and disabled physiotherapists generally, had improved in recent years. This is in direct contrast to the views expressed by the visually impaired physiotherapists in the first phase of the study where only 36.5 per cent felt welcomed by the professional body (see chapter 5). In the Equal Opportunities in Employment statement of the CSP it is stated:

> *The Chartered Society of Physiotherapy is committed to the view that the principles of equal opportunities in employment should be adhered to by all members of the Society. The Society recognises its responsibilities as a trade union and professional body to ensure that all members are treated equally and fairly. The Society pledges to support, defend and assist any member facing discrimination.*
> (Physiotherapy 1994c: 296)

Some of the physiotherapists mentioned the Disability Network which was initiated by the CSP in 1995 as a way of tackling discrimination within the profession. Equipment for visually impaired physiotherapists has also been installed at the headquarters of the CSP (Physiotherapy Frontline 1996). The majority of members of the Disability Network have visual impairments although some have hearing impairments, physical impairments and mental health problems. One of its tasks has been to review the accessibility of the CSP's literature for visually impaired physiotherapists

(Physiotherapy Frontline 1997c). Some of the physiotherapists saw changes such as this as resulting from various social pressures including the Disability Discrimination Act (1995). Lucy explained:

> *The Disability Discrimination Act has pressurised them and I think they have taken it on board very seriously...I think they're really trying to improve and instead of thinking of visually impaired physios as 'that little lot who were looked after by the RNIB' now we are part of them and they have taken that on. That has come about with the closure of the school, the Disability Discrimination Act and the general change of attitudes within society and everything.*

Ben could also see improvements but felt that the CSP was merely doing what was expected of it:

> *I don't expect it's ever wanted us, it's tolerated us in the past, and as a body it does it's best to cater for us now with offering to put certain information into braille and on tape...they're doing what is expected of them but I'm sure if we all went away there wouldn't be anybody who cried...we deflate their ego, there's still a bit of that mentality about.*

The resentment and hostility which is sometimes shown towards disabled people (Morris 1991, French et al 1997) was also discussed by George a physiotherapist interviewed in the first phase of the study:

> *Often there is an air of 'I feel very proud of this profession, and I do very complicated things, so how on earth can someone without sight do it too?'...it deflates their ego, it's an imperious attitude, a sense of jealousy. I found it when I was a superintendent and someone said to me 'This is an easy job, the department runs itself'.*

Robert who, at the time of the second interview was vice-chair of council of the CSP, believes he may have had some influence in bringing about positive changes for visually impaired physiotherapists:

> *I think that by someone like myself becoming involved in there hopefully that will have been helpful for other people as well because actually being there and 'doing' they get to know what you need...we've just agreed that the journal should be available in alternative formats. I think that's because I'm in that situation, as the vice-chair of council, though a lot of people have been pushing. I've been able to push from inside...there's a lot of goodwill these days, I don't think it's like it was 20 or 30 years ago for you and I.*

Despite some reservations, the visually impaired physiotherapists believe that physiotherapy is still a suitable profession for them. What doubts they have appear to focus on particular branches of physiotherapy, such as intensive care and community work, which gives rise to particular barriers which are difficult, although not impossible, to dislodge.

There is considerable tension in what the physiotherapists say with regard to whether or not they should be expected to manage every aspect of the job. The need to be 'as good as', if not better, that non-disabled workers may be necessary in order for disabled people to find and retain employment. This is reflected both in government literature and in the comments of disabled people (see chapter 2 and 3). It can also be seen as part of the struggle of visually impaired people to remain in the physiotherapy profession at particular points in time (see chapter 4). Sharron said:

> *The problem is, if you start introducing exemptions, you will introduce more barriers and people won't be as ready to employ a partially sighted person if they feel they won't be able to do 'on-call' and this and that...it creates more of a barrier and more of a stigma...it's politically dangerous.*

Conclusion

Despite a worsening of certain barriers since the passing of the NHS and Community Care Act (1990), the responses of the visually impaired physiotherapists, though mixed, show high levels of job satisfaction. Many people have reached high positions within the physiotherapy profession, despite reporting difficulties with promotion, although some people have avoided promotion because of the barriers they encounter. The attitude of the CSP towards visually impaired physiotherapists was reported as greatly improved since the first phase of the study.

The visually impaired physiotherapists have clearly experienced a complex mixture of influences during their careers. In many ways the work has become more demanding and challenging with, for example, an increase in community work and administration. On the other hand these barriers have, to some extent, been offset by improvements in attitudes and behaviour towards disabled people helped, perhaps, by equal opportunity policies and the passing of the Disability Discrimination Act (1995). Some of the physiotherapists were, however, doubtful that physiotherapy would be a viable career for visually impaired people, particularly totally blind people, in the future. This was because they felt that the increased demands of the job out-weighed the improvements that had been made in terms of attitudes and legislation.

Chapter 9

Personal Narratives: Disabling Barriers – Enabling Contexts

This chapter will present short personal narratives of three of the visually impaired physiotherapists, two men and one woman, who took part in both phases of the study. The aim of this chapter is to draw out some of the subtle and complex points concerning barriers and coping strategies which were not included in the thematic analysis of the interviews. These include the use of different coping strategies in different situations, the specific barriers and advantages of working in particular fields, the complexities of managing relationships and asking for help, the interaction of internal and external coping strategies and the priority given to the removal of barriers in different situations.

Terry

Terry has been visually impaired from birth and describes himself as being partially sighted. He spent all his school-days in mainstream education where his needs were not addressed. He left school with no qualifications but gained 'O' and 'A' level GCEs at a special college of further education for visually impaired students. Terry commenced his physiotherapy education in 1982 at the age of 22.

Terry has had a wide variety of physiotherapy posts some of which have been short-term through a medical agency. He said:

> *I've done everything – general hospital, military hospital...social services (that wasn't my forte at all). Then I went to work for Shell in industry...That was fascinating but I was only on a short term contract. Then I went to the hospital for tropical diseases but that was a short term contract too. In between all that lot I've done various locum jobs for weeks or months. Then ended up here. Quite a combination, it hasn't followed any kind of rhyme or reason.*

At the time of the interview in the second phase of the study, Terry was working as a senior 1 physiotherapist in mental health where he had been for three years. He refers to mental health as his 'niche'. The post involves work in in-patient, out-patient and community settings.

Mental health is quite an unusual field of work for physiotherapists and does not feature strongly in undergraduate education. This has involved Terry in considerable additional study:

> I've done a one year post-graduate diploma in supervision and counselling which is very helpful in doing this job...it was hard work because a lot of people who did that course came from mental health backgrounds...I also did a diploma in the theory and practice of group work which was absolutely fascinating...None of that, of course, we ever did at college.

In his interviews Terry described considerable problems with accessing information, including unpleasant symptoms such as headaches, and yet he was prepared to undertake a great deal of study in order to follow his chosen field of physiotherapy. This illustrates that visually impaired physiotherapists are prepared to surmount considerable barriers in order to achieve their aspirations and that visual impairment is only one attribute of the individual. The avoidance of disabling barriers, at the expense of achieving particular goals, is not always a major priority.

Terry found that his chosen field of physiotherapy posed particular problems for him as a visually impaired person. One problem, which he feels is made worse by visual impairment, is the threat of violence when he visits patients or clients at home:

> Patients with mental health problems are very unpredictable depending sometimes on whether they've been taking their medication or not...There was one particular incident where this chap had florid psychosis...he'd dislocated his knee cap and he'd been using a broom, turned up-side-down, to walk with – a bit like Long John Silver!...He became very abusive and chased me out of the house with this stick. He had a dislocated knee, but otherwise he probably would have brained me with it...You use your instinct much more than your vision if someone means you harm but you can pick up more quickly on what's going on if you can see.

Terry also finds the tendency of some depressed people to live in a darkened room problematic:

> Adjusting to the light is often tricky...Often you find that, if people are having a breakdown, they like to be shut in a very dark room. If I've come in from the outside it takes me ages to adjust. Quite often I walk into a room and I just stand there and they say 'Would you like to sit?' and I say 'I don't see very well, where would you like me to sit?'. But it works out all right.

Because of his interest in mental health Terry has not allowed these problems to deter him.

As well as focusing on difficulties, he also pointed out a very personal way in which his patients and clients have helped him as a disabled person:

> *I've learned such a lot about myself since being here...I've learned to be a lot more 'up-front' about my own visual impairment...what I find with the patients here is that they say exactly what's going on. I had a patient on the ward who said 'Can't you see properly? So I said 'I don't see at all well, I've got an eye condition'...And they all remember, they come up ever so close and say 'How you doing? Remember me?'. It's interesting that they are very much more 'up-front' and much more able to take it on board, there's none of the subtleties and nuances that you might expect...It's enabled me to be much more open about it.*

Despite the enthusiasm he shows for his work Terry is frustrated that there are so few opportunities for career advancement in the clinical grades. He hints that he might have changed his profession if there had been more opportunities:

> *I'm disappointed that there isn't greater opportunity within the field of physio to move on and go up as a clinician. I'm at the top end of the Senior 1 scale and have nowhere to go...People can become a Senior 1 very quickly and then where do you go?...I wish more opportunities in life were open to us. It really pleases me when I hear of someone who is visually impaired doing something unusual, going beyond the realms of what most people think we can manage.*

Like many physiotherapists, particularly the men, Terry supplements his income with part-time private practice.

Hilary

Hilary, who is a guide dog user, describes herself as having minimal sight. Hilary became visually impaired suddenly at the age of 22 after working as a Registered Mental Nurse for just one year. She wanted to continue working as a nurse but was not permitted to do so:

> *I decided to do my general State Registered training and just about a week before I started that I detached the retina of the right eye. I felt that I could go back to psychiatric nursing...but the hospital didn't so I had to leave. I did some voluntary work there for a time, they were quite happy for me to do that but they didn't want to pay me. I tried to be persuasive by demonstrating that I could do it by doing the voluntary work...but as far as they were concerned they were not able to take me on so in the end I admitted defeat.*

Hilary has always felt that this decision was wrong:

> *I can see the reasons why they were apprehensive. It was a psychiatric hospital and obviously you come across people who can be aggressive and being visually handicapped is probably not something one would expect to see in a staff member...but I felt that wasn't a good enough reason.*

It is not an unusual experience for people to lose their jobs with the onset of visual impairment (RNIB 1996a) or with the onset of impairment generally (Burchardt 2000).

Hilary went to a residential rehabilitation centre run by the RNIB when she first lost her sight and subsequently worked as an audio-typist:

> *When it first happened I went to Torquay to be assessed for 13 weeks and I managed to stick it out for five. It was the most horrendous experience of my life...I didn't like the institutionalisation as it was at that time...But I got some useful things out of it as I learned the keyboard and I learned braille. I then did an audio typing job...in the social services department and fortunately the standard they wanted was low – I wasn't very good...Then I worked in an insurance company for three years until I was able to move away from Bristol. I then had a choice between physiotherapy and social work. I was offered a place at Bristol Polytechnic for their two year social work course and I was also offered a place at the North London School and I chose physiotherapy.*

Hilary commenced her physiotherapy education in 1976 at the age of 26. She has specialised in out-patient work and management. Her current job involves her in management for a third of her time. Hilary finds that management has certain advantages for her as a visually impaired person:

> *I think it's much easier when you have control. It's much easier if you're the boss, you can plan what you do and you can delegate the rest...It's much easier than having to adjust to other people's policies and procedures.*

This shows the importance of the employee's position in the organisational hierarchy with regard to the removal of disabling barriers.

In the early part of her career Hilary spent two years working in the field of mental health as a senior physiotherapist:

> *They were desperate for someone. Physiotherapy hadn't previously been established in psychiatry – this was in 1982. There was a great reluctance on the part of most staff to move into that speciality. I didn't have any problems (getting the job) at all...It was comparatively easy for me because it was an environment I was very used to...I never got into a situation that I couldn't handle.*

It is ironic that Hilary should have been accepted so willingly as a physiotherapist in the mental health field but rejected as a nurse. As she suggests, this may be because mental health is not a popular area of physiotherapy practice. As noted in chapter 2, during times of staff shortages, for example during the First and Second World Wars, disabled people were able to find work much more easily (Humphries and Gordon 1992). It may also indicate a cultural change as considerable time had passed between her rejection as a nurse and her acceptance as a physiotherapist.

Hilary, who has a BA degree from the Open University, has experienced barriers and discrimination in post-graduate education particularly with regard to courses run by the Association of Manipulative Physiotherapists. This is interesting as manipulation is usually regarded as a skill which poses no problems for visually impaired people. Hilary explained the resistance in terms of factors other than visual impairment:

...I think it's partly to do with their culture...I think they wanted people who were seen to be top class practitioners and perhaps a visual impairment doesn't always give that impression initially.

This suggests that people respond to the 'aesthetics' of impairment (how it looks) rather than considering the functional limitations to which it may give rise and how any disabling barriers could be removed (Hahn 1990, Barnes et al 1998, Swain and French 1998).

Hilary's main coping strategy is openness and assertion:

You have to take control of the situation, to take the lead on it, because I think people who haven't encountered visual impairment before feel a bit uncomfortable and not very confident about what they should and shouldn't do. I've always found that most people like a little bit of guidance.

This indicates that visually impaired physiotherapists are expected to take the lead in the management of relationships with non-disabled people and cannot rely on others knowing very much about visual impairment.

Hilary users readers and computer technology to assist with administration but also adopts more personal coping strategies:

I use my memory much, much more, for example people are always saying 'how can you remember all the telephone numbers?'. Well, it's obvious why you do if you are visually impaired, because it takes you such a long time to look them up.

This illustrates that technical equipment does not entirely resolve the barrier of access to information and that visually impaired physiotherapists still use individual coping strategies to supplement different types of assistance. It was noted in chapters 6 and 7 that an excessive reliance on individual strategies, such as memory, is exhausting and stressful.

Robert

Robert describes himself as having minimum sight. He spent his schooldays in residential schools for blind children but was not, at the time, selected for a place at the grammar school for blind boys. Like Terry, Robert went to a college of further education for visually impaired students on leaving school where he gained qualifications in braille shorthand typing. The college did not offer GCE 'O' levels so he studied for these in the evening at a mainstream college. He worked for a short time in an office while he continued to study for his GCE 'O' levels. Like Hilary he viewed office work merely as a stepping stone towards another career. He said:

> *Office work was a stop gap, it wasn't something that I planned to get into, it was a convenient way of earning my living while doing a few other qualifications before deciding what I wanted to do. I was quite interested in the possibility of teaching, I wanted a job where I would contact the public in one way or another. I applied to a college in Bristol...but they saw too many problems from a visual point of view so it didn't progress any further.*

Robert's desire to teach was, therefore, denied. It is interesting to note the contrast between the educational experiences of Robert and Terry. Terry left mainstream education with no academic qualifications, which he subsequently acquired in a special college of further education, and Robert left special school with no academic qualifications which he subsequently acquired at a mainstream college.

Robert commenced his physiotherapy education at the RNIB School of Physiotherapy in 1968 at the age of 20. He has worked in hospital settings and, like Hilary, has mainly specialised in out-patient work and management. He did, however, work for several years on the wards which included neurology, neurosurgery and a cardio-thoracic unit, which involved intensive care, as a senior physiotherapist. Talking of work in intensive care, he said:

> *I thoroughly enjoyed it and had no problems from a visual point of view, the staff were very good, very helpful...I can't understand why blind people would find it difficult to be honest. The geography was straightforward, the conditions were easy enough to understand.*

Very many of the visually impaired physiotherapists expressed great concern about working in intensive care units (see chapter 7). Robert's comments illustrate, therefore, that barriers are not always absolute but are perceived and appraised by each individual and may vary according to the person's temperament, experience and wider contextual factors such as the support they receive.

A few years after qualifying as a physiotherapist Robert approached two mainstream schools of physiotherapy about the possibility of undertaking the Teacher of Physiotherapy Diploma which was offered jointly by the CSP and the North London Polytechnic. He was turned down by both schools of physiotherapy on the grounds of visual impairment and as he did not want to train at the RNIB School of Physiotherapy he abandoned the idea. His attempt to enter teaching within a mainstream setting was, therefore, denied yet again:

> *I applied when I was working at a teaching hospital and my application was quite sympathetically viewed but the Principal of the training school thought it would be better for me to go to the school for visually handicapped physios to do the training there...He felt that the problems might have been eased by working in an environment where they were used to working with visually handicapped students...at the time I wasn't particularly impressed with that sort of attitude.*

Robert's experience also indicates that the existence of a special facility may inhibit inclusion elsewhere.

Robert thought of going into private practice but, despite his interest in out-patient work, he did not feel it would suit him:

> *I felt it was too isolated for me. I'm also philosophically very much in favour of the NHS...I need the stimulation of other people around.*

This shows that visual impairment interacts with all other attributes of the person. It was found in the first phase of the study that some of the visually impaired physiotherapists, particularly the men, went into private practice, partly as a way of avoiding barriers, but Robert felt that this was not the right option for him because of his out-going personality and his commitment to the NHS.

Since 1983 Robert has been a full-time manager. He has reached the highest managerial post available to him as a physiotherapist and manages several occupational groups within various hospitals over a wide area. Talking of his promotion, Robert said:

> *I've been prepared to move around for the jobs I've wanted...the idea of lots of paper work can frighten your employers about how you can cope. Certainly for district posts I had to go through several interviews in several places before being appointed to the present one...but I know people with no sight problems who applied for more posts than I did.*

Robert experienced sexist attitudes in the early years of his career when trying to get promotion. He believes that physiotherapy is still a female dominated profession but realises that many of the managerial posts are occupied by men. This he refers to as 'a bit of a paradox, a contradiction'. The CSP (1996), in their survey on equal opportunities, found that far more men than women reported discrimination of various kinds, including discrimination associated with promotion, and yet men are heavily over-represented in the top management grades.

Robert has a BA degree from the Open University and an M.Phil in Social Policy and Administration from the University of Kent. At the time of the second interview he was working towards a PhD on 'Computerised Information Systems as a Management Tool' which he completed successfully in 2000.

Robert has, for many years undertaken a great deal of work for the CSP. He said:

> I was elected in 1983 so I've been on all sorts of committees as an elected member of council...industrial relations, service management, information systems. I was elected vice-chair of the council in 1995, that's a two year term...and then I can either stand to go on the chair of council or not. The likelihood is that I will.

(Robert was subsequently elected chair of the CSP council.)

In his position as a manager Robert is in a position to recruit staff. He has a very positive attitude towards the employment of visually impaired physiotherapists:

> We have a visually impaired member of staff...They are just as good, competent physios, they are not a problem at all...I would make sure, well do my best, that they had all the necessary facilities to do the job properly. With P... I made sure that the PACT (Placement, Assessment and counselling Team) people were involved to get her various pieces of equipment she needed...Having said that, at the end of the day they've got to do the job.

Talking of whether or not visually impaired physiotherapists should do intensive care, he said:

> I wouldn't force the issue...I would give fair weight to their feelings. If they didn't feel competent the chances are they might not be. So you might try them out, give them a bit of encouragement, perhaps assign a senior member of staff to oversee them a bit, and if it wasn't working out I would say 'This is not necessarily an area that we need to put you into'...There's so much flexibility that, well, why would I want to be difficult?

Robert's positive attitude towards visually impaired physiotherapists suggests that their situation might improve if more visually impaired people were in top management positions and had influential positions within the CSP.

Robert's major coping strategy is to be open and assertive regarding his needs. He said, 'I've always had to be prepared to ask for help, but that doesn't bother me, I'll ask anybody'. Like, Hilary, he also commented on the usefulness of his good memory:

I'm fortunate to have a good memory...it hasn't been a conscious strategy. I think I may just be lucky. I only have to read things once and it's in.

Like Hilary, Robert believes that his role as a senior manager has enabled him to avoid many employment barriers. He can, for example, delegate work, and his secretary assists him to minimise the barriers of administration.

Conclusion

These three short personal narratives illustrate how the disabling barriers visually impaired physiotherapists encounter, as well as the coping strategies they adopt, are modified according to many complex, interacting factors. These include the position the physiotherapist holds within the organisation (with those in higher positions having more choice and control) and the personality and aspirations of the individual person.

The barriers encountered are sometimes impenetrable (as in the case of Robert's desire to teach in a mainstream setting and Hilary's wish to continue nursing) but this too is dependent on the prevailing attitudes of the time and such factors as staff shortages. Some of the areas where the physiotherapists had worked may be thought by some to be unsuitable (for example intensive care and mental health) but any difficulties there are may be offset by various enabling factors, or the individual physiotherapist may simply not perceive the situation in terms of barriers, or the avoidance of barriers may not be a priority in terms of his or her overall goals and aspirations.

PART 3

OVERVIEW AND CONCLUDING COMMENTS

Chapter 10

Discussion and Conclusion

Some discussion of the findings of this study have been presented in chapters 4 to 9. In this chapter some over-arching themes will be discussed and the substantive findings of the research will be reiterated. Areas where the study has provided new insights will be highlighted and the chapter will conclude with suggestions for further research and the implications of the study for the education and employment of visually impaired physiotherapists and disabled people generally.

Substantive Findings

Different Characteristics of the Two Research Samples

The comparative study of visually impaired and sighted physiotherapists (see chapter 5) illustrates that the two samples are different in many ways other than visual impairment. There are large differences, for example, in the age and gender balance as well as differences in social background. These dissimilarities make interpretation of difference, with regard to many aspects of employment, problematic as it cannot be assumed to be the result of visual impairment alone. The differences between the two samples are, however, interesting in their own right and suggest, for example, that social background is not a determinant of success as a physiotherapist. The large number of male visually impaired physiotherapists, in what is still predominantly a female profession, indicates restriction in choice of occupation for visually impaired people which was commented upon by both the male and female research respondents.

The age and gender differences may have had an effect on work speciality and promotion. In the first phase of the study, for example, it was found that a high proportion of visually impaired men were in private practice. Although some of the physiotherapists related this to a wish to create an environment free of barriers, they also spoke of the necessity to support their families and their desire for a higher salary than the NHS would provide.

The age difference between the two samples may have had an effect on work speciality, promotion and job satisfaction. The high job satisfaction of the visually impaired physiotherapists may also have been influenced, to some degree, by their knowledge that the majority of visually impaired people of working age are unemployed. The work grades of the visually impaired physiotherapists are very similar to those of the sighted physiotherapists. This may, however, have been influenced by the fact that the visually impaired sample contain a far greater proportion of men, who may find promotion easier than female physiotherapists, and that they are older and may, therefore, have had more time to rise up the occupational hierarchy.

The attitudinal differences between the two samples, for example regarding the inclusion of visually impaired physiotherapists in mainstream physiotherapy education (where the sighted sample were more positive), may also reflect age and gender differences at least in part. It may also be the case that the sighted physiotherapists were attempting to avoid prejudice in the absence of sufficient understanding or experience of the substantial difficulties of inclusive education for visually impaired physiotherapists. Direct experience may, therefore, be an important factor, as well as gender and age, in the attitudes of visually impaired physiotherapists.

Major Barriers

Seven major barriers in the working lives of the visually impaired physiotherapists emerged in the study. These barriers concerned administration, transport, medical equipment, post-registration education, mobility (particularly in wards and intensive care units), meetings and the attitudes and behaviour of employers and colleagues. These barriers clearly relate to the social model of disability and the concept of institutional discrimination (Oliver 1990, Swain et al 1998). Problems with administrative work could, for example, be made worse by the unhelpful attitudes and behaviour of colleagues, by having to process it too quickly or by the need to cope without appropriate equipment or help. The barriers also show how wider factors, such as transport, can impact on the ability of disabled people to work or to have choice of employment. Barriers are, therefore, interwoven and cannot be easily dismantled piece by piece. This issue was examined in relation to institutional discrimination (see chapter 1) and will be explored later in this chapter.

The ways in which the barriers were experienced and their severity varied according to many factors including the physiotherapists' degree of vision, their place of employment, their speciality, their position within the occupational hierarchy and personality factors. Administration tended, for example, to be a greater barrier for those physiotherapists who were unable to read print than for those who could, although those in top managerial posts were more likely to be given the services of a secretary which minimised the barriers regardless of the physiotherapist's level of sight.

The blind physiotherapists sometimes appeared to be given more help than those with some sight as their impairment is more obvious to patients, clients and colleagues. These examples indicate, in support of the social model of disability and the concept of institutional discrimination, that the degree of disability experienced varies according to environmental circumstances and that there is no simple causal connection between impairment and disability. The degree of impairment does, however, affect the type of barriers that are encountered.

Although many of the barriers were embedded within organisational practices and structures, they were sometimes both created and removed according to a particular manager's or colleague's attitude and behaviour. This indicates that some improvement can be made by individuals even though institutional discrimination, in terms of environmental and structural barriers, remains intact. Hospital Trusts also responded very differently to visually impaired physiotherapists with one, for example, providing a visually impaired manager with a car and a person to drive it, while another relocated a visually impaired manager to a site without convenient public transport and offered no assistance (see chapter 7). Any assistance or consideration the physiotherapists received overall was, therefore, highly erratic. It remains to be seen how helpful the employment section of the Disability Discrimination Act (1995) will be.

The physiotherapists did not necessarily react in the same way to apparently similar barriers. Some physiotherapists, for example, spoke of how enabling they found technology whereas others found it daunting and disabling. Training with specialised computer technology, for example, is limited but, whereas some physiotherapists perceived this as an extreme barrier, others were undaunted and managed to teach themselves. In some instances their views appeared to relate to how psychologically comfortable, as individuals, they felt with new technology. Gender may also have been a factor as the male physiotherapists seemed more at ease with technology although the numbers are too small to verify this impression. It is also possible that visually impaired physiotherapists younger than those who took part in this study, may feel more at ease with technology.

The barriers in the second phase of the study were very similar to those which were identified in the first phase. Many physiotherapists perceived their situation to be getting worse with more administration, more community work, less accessible equipment and an increased pace of work with greater pressure. Some physiotherapists related this to changes in the NHS following the NHS and Community care Act (1990) although similar concerns were expressed in the first phase of the study before this Act was passed. This suggests that the legislation may have been a response to policy and practice which was already occurring in the 1980s. Despite these problems most visually impaired physiotherapists reported a high degree of job satisfaction.

One notable improvement mentioned by the physiotherapists was the attitude of the CSP toward them which is now far more responsive to visually impaired physiotherapists as well as other minority groups within the profession (see chapter 7). The physiotherapists also appeared to experience less overt prejudice and discrimination than at earlier phases of their careers (see chapters 4 to 9). It is disturbing to find, however, that the barriers which were identified in the first phase of the study were largely in place in the second phase. The physiotherapists were, for example, less likely to be refused entry to post-registration education but were still frequently compelled to cope with inaccessible teaching and learning methods.

Some of the visually impaired physiotherapists mentioned internal barriers such as embarrassment and feelings of inadequacy. These feelings could, for example, deter them from seeking promotion or asking for help on a course. Although barriers of this type are not emphasised in the social model of disability, they have been discussed within the disabled people's movement especially by disabled women (see chapter 1) who have sought to extend the social model of disability by taking such factors into account. These negative feelings may be the result of the ways in which the visually impaired physiotherapists are treated, or have been treated, as disabled people in the past (internal oppression), or they may be a response to dealing constantly with disabling barriers without support which may lower self-esteem (Simkiss et al 1998).

Most of the visually impaired physiotherapists who mentioned these feelings related them, at least in part, to childhood experiences of bullying, being unacceptable to others as disabled people, and having their visual impairments minimised or denied. The reporting of feelings such as embarrassment and inadequacy were more common among the female physiotherapists although the numbers are too small to verify the significance of this.

The barriers the visually impaired physiotherapists experienced at work are similar to those experienced by other disabled people (Barnes et al 1998) and other disabled health and welfare workers (French 1988) as highlighted in chapters 2 and 3. Most of the physiotherapists viewed the problems they encountered in terms of external barriers, rather than in terms of impairment, which tallies with the social model of disability and the concept of institutional discrimination (see chapter 1).

Some of the visually impaired physiotherapists did, however, mention unpleasant symptoms relating to impairment, for example headaches, and some were of the opinion that physiotherapy had become too difficult, within the NHS, for totally blind people, because of their blindness. This was related, however, to the expectation that blind physiotherapists should be equally as versatile as sighted physiotherapists. Others spoke about barriers which cannot readily be changed through social manipulation, such as the inability to recognise people or to perceive non-verbal language. Hughes and Paterson suggest that disabled people encounter impairment and disability 'as part of a complex interpenetration of oppression and affliction' (1997: 335). This appears to be the case for some of the visually impaired physiotherapists in this study who spoke in terms both of impairment and disabling barriers.

This study illustrates the power of external barriers to shape the working lives of visually impaired physiotherapists and the importance of the social model of disability and the concept of institutional discrimination in explaining disability at work. The physiotherapists did, however, discuss internal barriers and aspects of impairment which are not readily overcome, minimised or managed by altering the environment. The study also illustrates that visual impairment is just one attribute of the individual, which interacts with all other attributes, and that what one person perceives as a barrier may not be perceived as a barrier by another person with a similar impairment.

Major Coping Strategies

Various coping strategies to overcome, minimise or manage the barriers encountered were highlighted by the visually impaired physiotherapists. These included asking for help of colleagues, patients and clients, using specialised equipment and readers provided by the Access to Work scheme, working longer hours, using taxis and hospital transport, adapting equipment, and personal strategies such as the use of echo location to aid mobility, concentration, and developing a good memory.

Asking help of colleagues was a major coping strategy although many physiotherapists related incidents of colleagues' attitudes and behaviour producing barriers. The erosion of the Access to Work scheme, which the majority of the physiotherapists used, was also viewed as a barrier. This indicates that visually impaired physiotherapists lack rights at work and are dependent on the attitudes and behaviour of colleagues and on government policy which varies and is beyond their control.

Four major coping strategies were highlighted by the visually impaired physiotherapists: openness and assertion; minimisation of disability; compensation; and avoidance of difficulties (see chapter 7). The majority of the physiotherapists were open about disability and asked for what they needed. Many said that this had become easier with age and with a more senior position. A minority of the physiotherapists spoke of minimising or 'playing down' their disability. This strategy appeared to be associated with feelings of insecurity and was more common among those physiotherapists with some sight where 'passing' as a sighted person was more feasible (Goffman 1968, French 1997c). Minimising disability is not an irrational or pathological act. The research by Fry (1986) cited in chapter 2 illustrates the devastating consequences that revealing disability can have. Attempting to compensate for disability, by, for example, working longer hours or rarely taking sick leave, and avoiding areas of difficulty, for example intensive care, were also common coping strategies among the physiotherapists.

The coping strategies used by the visually impaired physiotherapists were not constant but varied according to the social context. The physiotherapists were more likely to be open about disability, for example, if their employers and colleagues were supportive or if they were in a senior position. In addition, some of the physiotherapists said that they had become more assertive and open with age, probably as a result of becoming more confident. The degree of impairment also had an effect on the coping strategies adopted. Those physiotherapists with some sight, for example, were more able to minimise disability than blind physiotherapists and the blind physiotherapists were more dependent on internal strategies such as echo location and memory.

Insights From the Study

Visually impaired physiotherapists are a unique group of employees in Britain who have not been studied extensively before. It was noted in chapter 4 that the inclusion of visually impaired people within the physiotherapy profession may be regarded as an historical accident inasmuch as physiotherapy originates from massage which visually impaired people traditionally practised. It is unlikely that physiotherapy would be considered a suitable occupation for visually impaired people today (at least by sighted people) as it requires many activities where sight may be thought essential. This study shows that visually impaired people can work successfully in, and contribute significantly towards, a profession with many potential barriers and one in which high levels of stress are recognised (Broom and Williams 1996). The study thus throws doubt upon 'taken for granted' assumptions about what work visually impaired people, and other disabled people, can and cannot do.

There has been very little research on disabled employees from the perspective of the employees themselves (Barnes et al 1998). Although this study focuses upon a very specific group, it can be regarded as a case study of the barriers that visually impaired people, and disabled people generally, experience at work and the ways in which they overcome, minimise or manage them. All of the major barriers identified, for example transport and access to information, relate to other visually impaired people and to many other disabled people.

This study extends the social model of disability by analysing the complexity of disabling barriers. There is considerable agreement among the visually impaired physiotherapists on what constitutes barriers and yet it is also clear that barriers are perceived, appraised and experienced differently according to such factors as personality, age, degree of visual impairment, position in the occupational hierarchy, and whether or not the person feels supported by employers and colleagues. It may also be the case that gender and the social background and experience of the individual influences the ways in which barriers are perceived, experienced and managed.

On occasions these contextual and individual factors can modify barriers directly, for example the visually impaired managers had the power to modify their environments and blind physiotherapists found help more forthcoming on some occasions than physiotherapists with some sight. It is also the case, however, that visually impaired physiotherapists, in a very similar situation, sometimes perceive, appraise and act upon barriers differently, for example those relating to intensive care and technology. This shows that barriers are not necessarily absolute, but exist within a social context and can be modified by factors within that context. It also shows that visual impairment is just one attribute of the person which interacts with all other attributes when potential barriers are appraised.

The removal of disabling barriers is frequently regarded in a somewhat simplistic way. It may be thought, for example that by giving a visually impaired person a document in large print or braille the barrier of standard print will be entirely removed. This study indicates, however, that the removal of disabling barriers is far more complex. Despite sophisticated technology, for example, the visually impaired physiotherapists were still slower than their colleagues and were compelled to work longer hours to hold down their jobs. This indicates that in order to remove disabling barriers structural changes, as well as environmental changes, need to be made, for example allowing visually impaired people to do less administration or giving them more time in the working day to do it.

This is not without problems, however, as it may, in turn. lead to an increase in attitudinal barriers among colleagues although some of the visually impaired physiotherapists had successfully negotiated informal arrangements whereby they did do less administration or were exempt from work in intensive care units. Some of the physiotherapists were dubious about introducing 'special arrangements' with one describing it as 'politically dangerous'. It was noted in chapter 4 that visually impaired physiotherapists have had a struggle over the century to retain their position within the physiotherapy profession and have been obliged to find ways of coping with the work, for example by the adaptation of equipment. There appears to have been a drive to minimise the difference between sighted and visually impaired physiotherapists in order for visually impaired physiotherapists to be accepted within the profession. The need to maintain a competent image may also inhibit the removal of disabling barriers.

Reliance on internal strategies, such as echo location, memory and concentration would seem to go against the spirit of the social model of disability and the concept of institutional discrimination where it is proposed that disability is located within society and should, therefore, be removed by society. This study shows that the visually impaired physiotherapists were strongly orientated to removing external barriers, rather than trying to change themselves. When they spoke about reliance on internal strategies they frequently pointed out how stressful and exhausting it was. They did, however, use a combination of strategies to overcome, minimise or manage barriers. Hilary, for example, spoke of developing a good memory for telephone numbers as it was much quicker than retrieving them through her computer equipment. It seems likely that the removal of disabling barriers will need to be considerably extended before visually impaired physiotherapists can stop relying on internal strategies. It may also be the case that, even within an environment free of barriers, these strategies would still develop in the absence of sight.

Advocates of the social model of disability have tended to evade discussion of impairment and the particular disabling barriers that people with different impairments experience. This study makes it clear, however, that even people with the same impairment label (in this case visual impairment) experience different barriers according to the type and degree of impairment. It has been noted in this study, for example, that blind physiotherapists experience more mobility barriers than physiotherapists with some sight and that physiotherapists with some sight experience particular attitudinal barriers (with, for example, colleagues misunderstanding or disbelieving the severity of their impairments) which blind physiotherapists are less likely to experience. Colleagues appear to behave differently towards blind physiotherapists and physiotherapists with some sight, for example offering help more readily to blind physiotherapists but having less confidence in their ability to practise physiotherapy (see chapter 5). It would seem also that physiotherapists with some sight are more likely, and in a better position, to use 'minimisation' as a coping strategy.

This study indicates, particularly from the personal narratives, that the removal of disabling barriers is not always a top priority of the visually impaired physiotherapists. Like many people, the visually impaired physiotherapists have major goals and aspirations within their working lives which they attempt to pursue, according to their personalities and interests, regardless of barriers. Not all of the blind physiotherapists, for example, worked in private practice although this, from the point of view of barrier removal, would be the obvious thing to do. Reasons such as 'believing in the NHS' and not wanting to work alone were given for not opting for maximum barrier removal.

Recommendations for Practice and Further Research

Many of the physiotherapists in the second phase of the study spoke of the attempts being made by the CSP to remove disabling barriers and to meet their needs. This process has, however, only just begun. This study will provide useful information, directly from visually impaired physiotherapists, about the barriers they experience at work and how these barriers may be removed. It will be useful to the professional body and to any employer interested in removing the barriers visually impaired physiotherapists encounter. It will also be a useful source of information for policy makers and employers of other visually impaired and disabled people who wish to analyse employment barriers and their removal. The recent passing of the Disability Discrimination Act (1995), despite its weaknesses (see chapter 2), has made the issue of disabling barriers an urgent reality for many employers.

The research on disabled people and employment, from the viewpoint of disabled people themselves, is sparse (Barnes et al 1998) as is research which focuses on external barriers (Zarb 1995b). More research is needed in other employment settings to provide a comprehensive picture of the barriers visually impaired and other disabled people face and the strategies used to overcome, minimise or manage them. This study highlights tremendous variation from one employer to another and gives instances of both good and bad practice. Other issues which have been outside the scope of this study also deserves attention, for example. the different experiences of disabled male and female employees, the employment experiences of disabled people from ethnic minorities, and the changing experiences of disabled employees as they grow older.

The removal of disabling barriers for visually impaired people is complex and depends, not only on the person concerned (his or her impairment, personality and aspirations) but also on the social context. It is important that visually impaired people are consulted about their requirements and that assumptions are not made on the basis of what another visually impaired person can and cannot do. This applies equally to other disabled people. The tendency to view the person's impairment as his or her 'master status' (Goffman 1968), obscuring all other characteristics, should also be avoided.

This study makes it clear that the assistance visually impaired physiotherapists receive is haphazard and dependent on many factors including their position within the hierarchy, the attitudes and behaviour of their employers and colleagues, and the particular Hospital Trust in which they work. This erratic situation can lead to stress and may inhibit some visually impaired physiotherapists from changing jobs or seeking promotion. It is clear that, despite existing legislation and equal opportunity policies, visually impaired physiotherapists are still substantially disadvantaged at work.

With the passing of the Disability Discrimination Act (1995) the rights of disabled employees are beginning to be addressed. This Act, though weak, can be used by visually impaired physiotherapists and other disabled employees to serve as a framework for the removal of barriers. The Act stipulates, for example, that premises are adjusted, that training is arranged and that equipment is modified for disabled workers. It also specifies that disabled workers should be treated flexibly and that work practices should be modified to accommodate them by, for example, allocating some of the disabled person's duties to another person or assigning a disabled person to a different place of work (see chapter 2). Requirements such as these, if taken seriously, could allow visually impaired physiotherapists to work flexibly within the NHS by, for example, avoiding areas which they find particularly difficult, such as work in intensive care units. This may reduce some of the pressure many visually impaired people feel to be proficient in all areas of physiotherapy. Dogma concerning what visually impaired people, and indeed all disabled people, can and cannot do must, however, be avoided.

Although the Disability Discrimination Act (1995) does not at present require the dismantling of disabling barriers in education, most post-registration education for physiotherapists is covered by the Act as in-service training is regarded as part of the physiotherapist's employment. Whatever the situation with regard to the Act, it is vitally important that disabling barriers are removed. The situation for visually impaired physiotherapists would be greatly improved by simple measures such as preparing handouts and book lists in advance, putting printed material into a suitable format, orientating the person to the venue, and assisting with transport. Some modifications may, however, take more thought. Visually impaired physiotherapists are likely, for example, to need more time to take notes or they may need to feel rather than watch a demonstration. This also applies to pre-registration education.

Most of the visually impaired physiotherapists in this study used the Access to Work scheme for equipment, readers and (occasionally) transport. Although there were criticisms of the scheme, particularly in terms of quality of service and training, most of the physiotherapists were positive about it and some were alarmed and outraged by the alterations to the scheme requiring the employer to bear some of the cost. This study suggests that the Access to Work scheme should be extended and strengthened, rather than dismantled, and that it should be used flexibly to meet the needs of individual people.

Conclusion

This study shows that negative and positive factors have co-existed within the careers of visually impaired physiotherapists both to create and to remove barriers. A greater emphasis on equal opportunity policies and the passing of the Disability Discrimination Act (1995) may have helped to create a more favourable attitudinal climate but, at the same time, changes in working practice within the NHS, brought about partly by the NHS and Community Care Act (1990), have made the situation more difficult for many visually impaired physiotherapists. Thus changes in health and disability legislation, policy, practice, and values, have had an impact upon the working lives of visually impaired physiotherapists in diverse and unexpected ways.

This study shows that, although external barriers can, in some instances, be removed, the barriers experienced by visually impaired physiotherapists are still viewed within organisations largely as an individual problem. Enabling practices are not built into the organisational structure of the NHS and visually impaired physiotherapists are left largely to find their own solutions to what are regarded as 'their' problems. Institutional discrimination has not, therefore, been tackled in any fundamental way. Change has been very slow and many of the visually impaired physiotherapists report problems at work that they were experiencing ten or more years ago. Although this research cannot be generalised automatically to other disabled people, the picture presented of numerous barriers, as well as the coping strategies employed to overcome, minimise or manage them, tallies with other research on disabled people and employment and disabled health and welfare workers (see French 1988, Barnes et al 1998, Simkiss et al 1998, Burchardt 2000).

The ways in which minority and oppressed groups have been treated throughout history has been diverse and the path of improvement has not been straightforward. This can be illustrated at various points within this study, particularly in relation to the attitudes and behaviour of specific individuals. Some non-disabled people, for example, were positive and helpful towards visually impaired physiotherapists many years ago while others are less than helpful today. In the early years of physiotherapy education (from 1900 to 1915) Dr. Fletcher Little integrated visually impaired students into his mainstream school of massage (see chapter 4). The concept of integrated education for visually impaired people is, therefore, far from new. In the 1950s two electrotherapy manufacturers built features into their machines so that visually impaired physiotherapists could use them (see chapter 7). This, even today, in a highly unusual response. Both of these examples illustrate attempts, decades ago, to remove disabling barriers.

Visually impaired physiotherapists have succeeded in the physiotherapy profession as clinicians, managers, lecturers and private practitioners. They have done so despite numerous barriers although they have always had many allies within the profession and enormous support from patients and clients. The serious shortage of physiotherapists which has, and does, bedevil the NHS may also have played its part in assisting visually impaired physiotherapists to find work and gain promotion on a par with their sighted colleagues.

It is unclear from this study whether visually impaired physiotherapists experience fewer barriers than other disabled employees by virtue of the length of time they have spent within the profession. What is clear, however, is that their presence within the profession has not, of itself, been sufficient to dismantle all the disabling barriers they encounter. This would involve substantial changes at the structural, environmental and attitudinal level. Visually impaired people have been 'assimilated' into the physiotherapy profession (allowed to enter it as it stands) but have not been 'included' within it which would entail altering the environment and working practices to enable visually impaired physiotherapists to work to their full potential within a non-disabling environment.

Bibliography

Abberley, P. (1995), 'Disabling Ideology in Health and Welfare – The Case of Occupational Therapy', *Disability and Society*, Vol. 10, No. 2, pp. 221–232.

Abberley, P. (1996), 'Work, Utopia and Impairment', in L. Barton (ed), *Disability and Society: Emerging Issues and Insights*, Longman, London, pp. 61–79.

Abercrombie, N., Hill, S. and Turner, B. (1988), *Dictionary of Sociology*, Penguin Books, Harmondsworth.

Allen, M. and Birse, E. (1991), 'Stigma and Blindness', *Journal of Ophthalmic Nursing and Technology*, Vol. 10, No. 4, pp. 147–151.

Allen, T. and Thomas, A. (eds) (2000), *Poverty and Development: Into the 21st Century*, Oxford University Press, Oxford.

Apter, D. (1992), 'A Successful Competitive/Supportive Environment for People with Severe Visual Disabilities', *Journal of Vocational Rehabilitation*, Vol. 2, No. 1, pp. 21–27.

Argyle, M. (1988) *Bodily Communication* (2nd ed), Routledge, London.

Ash, A., Bellew, J., Davies, M., Newman, T. and Richardson, L. (1997), 'Everybody In? The Experience of Disabled Students in Further Education', *Disability and Society*, Vol. 12, No. 4, pp. 605–21.

Association of Blind Certified Masseurs (1905), Annual Report.

Association of Blind Certified Masseurs (1928), Annual Report.

Association of Blind Certified Masseurs (1931), Annual Report.

Association of Blind Certified Masseurs (1934), Annual Report.

Association of Blind Certified Masseurs (1936), Annual Report.

Association of Blind Chartered Physiotherapists and St. Dunstan's (Undated pamphlet).

Atkinson, D., McCarthy, M., Walmsley, J., Cooper, M., Rolph, S., Aspis, S., Barette, P., Coventry, M. and Ferris, G. (eds) (2000), *Good Times, Bad Times: Women with Learning Difficulties Telling Their Stories*, British Institute of Learning Disabilities, Kidderminster.

Atkinson, R.L., Atkinson, G.C., Smith, E.E. and Bem, D.J. (1993), *Introduction to Psychology* (11th ed), Harcourt Brace Jovanovich College Publishers, London.

Balser, R. and Harvey, B. (1993), 'Using Hospitals as Job Training and Employment Sites for People with Disabilities', *Journal of Vocational Rehabilitation*, Vol. 3, No. 4, pp. 56–60.

Barclay, J. (1994), *In Good Hands: The History of The Chartered Society of Physiotherapy, 1894–1994*, Butterworth-Heinemann, Oxford.

Barnes, C. (1991), *Disabled People in Britain and Discrimination: A Case for Anti-Discrimination Legislation*, The Hurst Company, London, in association with the British Council of Organisations of Disabled People.

Barnes, C. (1992), *Disabling Imagery and the Media*, Ryburn, Belper.

Barnes, C. (1996), 'Visual Impairment and Disability', in G. Hales (ed), *Beyond Disability: Towards an Enabling Society*, Sage, London, pp. 36–44.

Barnes, C. (1998), 'The Social Model of Disability: A Sociological Phenomenon Ignored By Sociologists', in T. Shakespeare (ed), *The Disability Reader: Social Science Perspectives*, Cassell, London, pp. 65–78.

Barnes, C. and Mercer, G. (eds) (1997), *Doing Disability Research*, The Disability Press, Leeds.

Barnes, H., Thornton, P. and Maynard Campbell, S. (1998), *Disabled People and Employment: A Review of Research and Development Work*, The Policy Press, Bristol.

Baron, S., Phillips, R. and Stalker, K. (1996), 'Barriers to Training for Disabled Social Work Students', *Disability and Society*, Vol. 11, No. 3, pp. 361–377.

Bennet, G. (1987), *The Wound of the Doctor*, Secker and Warburg, London.

Borland, J. and James, S. (1999), 'The Learning Experiences of Students with Disabilities in Higher Education: A Case Study of a UK University', *Disability and Society*, Vol. 14, No. 1, pp. 85–101.

Bourke, J. (1996), *Deconstructing the Male: Men's Bodies, Britain and the Great War*, Reaktion Books, London.

Bradfield, A.L. (1992), 'Environmental Assessment and Job Site Modification for People Who Are Visually Impaired', *Journal of Vocational Rehabilitation*, Vol. 2, No.1, pp. 39–45.

British Society of Audiology, *Employment and Training of Audiology Technicians* (undated), London.

Broom, J.P. and Williams, J. (1996), 'Occupational Stress and Neurological Rehabilitation Physiotherapists', *Physiotherapy*, Vol. 82, No.11, pp. 606–614.

Bruce, I., McKennell, A. and Walker, E. (1991), *Blind and Partially Sighted Adults in Britain: The RNIB Survey*, HMSO Publications, London.

Burchardt, T. (2000), *Enduring Economic Exclusion: Disabled People, Income and Work*, Joseph Rowntree Foundation, York.

Burnfield, A. (1985), *Multiple Sclerosis: A Personal Exploration*, Souvenir Press, London.

Campbell, J. and Oliver, M. (1996), *Disability Politics: Understanding Our Past, Changing our Future*, Routledge, London.

Casserley, C. (2000), Human Rights and Disability, *New Beacon*, Vol. 84, No. 990, pp. 32–33.

Chartered Society of Physiotherapy (1971a), *Minutes of the Chartered Society of Physiotherapy Council*, 26th May, London.

Chartered Society of Physiotherapy (1971b), *Inspectors' Report on the Royal National Institute for the Blind School of Physiotherapy*, 13th January, London.

Chartered Society of Physiotherapy (1975), *Modification in the Curriculum of Training for Visually Handicapped Students*, London.

Chartered Society of Physiotherapy (1984), *How to Become a Chartered Physiotherapist*, London.

Chartered Society of Physiotherapy (1994a), *Professional Development Diary* (2nd ed), London.

Chartered Society of Physiotherapy (1994b), *The History of the Chartered Society of Physiotherapy 1894–1994*, London (Pamphlet).

Chartered Society of Physiotherapy (1996), *Equal Opportunity Working Party: Survey of CSP Members*, London.

Chartered Society of Physiotherapy (1998), *Physiotherapy: A Career in a Caring Profession*, London.
Chinnery, B. (1990), 'Soapbox', *Social Work Today*, 17th May, p. 23.
Chinnery, B. (1991), 'Equal Opportunities for Disabled People in the Caring Professions: Window Dressing or Commitment?', *Disability Handicap and Society*, Vol. 6, No. 3, pp. 253–258.
Clarke, J. and Saraga, E. (1998), 'Introduction', in E. Saraga (ed), *Embodying the Social: Constructions of Difference*, Routledge, London, pp. 1–2.
College of Radiographers (1985), *Radiography – Your Career?*, London.
Colorez, A. and Geist, E.O. (1987), 'Rehabilitation vs General Employer Attitudes Towards Hiring Disabled Persons', *Journal of Rehabilitation*, Vol. 51, No. 2, pp. 44–47.
Cooke, C., Daone, L. and Morris, G. (2000), *Stop Press: How the Press Portrays Disabled People*, Scope, London.
Cooper, J. and Vernon, S. (1996), *Disability and the Law*, Jessica Kingsley Publishers, London.
Cooper, N., Stevenson, C. and Hale, G. (1996), 'The biopsychosocial model', in N. Cooper, C. Stevenson, and G. Hale (eds), *Integrating Perspectives on Health*, Open University Press, Buckingham, pp. 1–17.
Corbett, J. (1996), *Bad Mouthing: The Language of Special Needs*, The Falmer Press, London.
Corley, G., Robinson, D. and Lockett, S. (1989), *Partially Sighted Children*, NFER-Nelson Publishing Company Limited, Windsor.
Cornes, P. (1991), 'Impairment, Disability, Handicap and New Technology', in M. Oliver (ed), *Social Work, Disabled People and Disabling Environments*, Jessica Kingsley Publishers, London, pp. 98–114.
Craik, C. (1990), 'Disability Need Not be a Barrier to a Career in Occupational Therapy', *Contact*, Vol. 66, pp. 14–16.
Crow, L. (1996), 'Including all of our Lives: Renewing the Social Model of Disability', in J. Morris (ed), *Encounters with Strangers: Feminism and Disability*, The Women's Press, London, pp. 206–226.
Curtis, J., McGinty, J. and Maudslay, L. (1997), *Quality and Equality: Good Practice in Vocational Training for Visually Impaired People*, Royal Society for the Blind, London.
Davis, K. (1993a), 'On the Movement', in J. Swain, V. Finkelstein, S. French and M. Oliver (eds), *Disabling Barriers – Enabling Environments*, Sage, London, pp. 285–292.
Davis, K. (1993b), 'The Crafting of Good Clients', in J. Swain, V. Finkelstein, S. French and M. Oliver (eds), *Disabling Barriers – Enabling Environments*, Sage, London, pp. 197–200.
Davison, G.C. and Neale, J.M. (1990), *Abnormal Psychology* (5th ed), John Wiley and Sons, Chichester.
Dench, S., Meager, N. and Morris, S. (1996), '*The Recruitment and Retention of People with Disabilities*, Institute of Employment Studies, London.
Department of Employment (1990), *More Than Just A Symbol: A Message for Employers*, Employment Service, London.
Deshen, S. (1992), *Blind People*, State University of New York Press, New York.

Disability – Changing Practice (1990), Disability Equality Pack (K665x), Open University, Milton Keynes.

Dodds, A.G. (1993), *Rehabilitating Blind and Visually Impaired People*, Chapman and Hall, London.

Downs, C. (1999), 'Enhancing Interaction with People with Severe and Profound Learning Difficulties', in J. Swain and S. French (eds), *Therapy and Learning Difficulties: Advocacy, Participation and Partnership*, Butterworth-Heinemann, Oxford, pp. 299–311.

Doyle, B.J. (1996), *Disability The New Law*, Jordan's Publishing Limited, Bristol.

Duckett, P.S. (2000), 'Disabling Employment Interviews: Warfare to Work', *Disability and Society*, Vol. 15, No. 7, pp. 1019–1039.

Dyer, L. (1990), 'The Right to Work' (Draft copy of paper for 'Open Mind'), Cited in Barnes, C. (1991), *Disabled People in Britain and Discrimination: A Case for Anti-Discrimination Legislation*, Hurst and Company, London, in Association with the British Council of Organisations of Disabled People.

Edwards, K. (1986), *'Becoming a Speech Pathologist: My Struggle With the University'*, *The Braille Monitor*, July, pp. 307–311.

Elliott, D.L., Hanzlik, R. and Gliner, J.A. (1992), 'Attitudes of Occupational Therapy Personnel Towards Therapists with Disabilities', *Occupational Therapy Journal of Research*, Vol. 12, No. 5, pp. 259–277.

Farish, M., McPake, J., Powney, J. and Weiner, G. (1995), *Equal Opportunities in Colleges and Universities: Towards Better Practices*, The Society for Research into Higher Education and Open University Press, Buckingham.

Fernando, S. (1989), *Race and Culture in Psychiatry*, Routledge, London.

Finkelstein, V. (1981), 'To Deny or Not to Deny Disability', in A. Brechin, P. Liddiard and J. Swain (eds), *Handicap in a Social World*, Hodder and Stoughton, Sevenoaks, pp. 34–36.

Finkelstein, V. (1993), 'Disability: A Social Challenge or an Administrative Responsibility?' in J. Swain, V. Finkelstein, S. French and M. Oliver (eds), *Disabling Barriers – Enabling Environments*, Sage, London, pp. 34–43.

Finkelstein, V. (1998), 'Emancipating Disability Studies', in T. Shakespeare (ed), *The Disability Reader: Social Science Perspectives*, Cassell, London, pp. 28–49.

Finkelstein, V. and French, S. (1993), 'Towards a Psychology of Disability', in J. Swain, V. Finkelstein, S. French and M. Oliver (eds), *Disabling Barriers – Enabling Environments*, Sage, London, pp. 26–33.

Finkelstein, V. and Stuart, O. (1996), 'Developing New Services' in G. Hales (ed), *Beyond Disability: Towards an Enabling Society*, Sage, London, pp. 170–187.

Fishbein, M. and Ajken, I. (1975), *Belief, Attitude, Intention and Behaviour*, Addison-Wesley, Reading, Massachusetts.

Fletcher Little, J. (1904), 'Massage by the Blind', *The Blind*, Vol. 2, No. 46, pp. 144–148.

Foley, C. and Pratt, S. (1994), *Access Denied: Human Rights and Disabled People*, National Council for Civil Liberties, London.

French, S. (1986), *Handicapped People in the Health and Caring Professions – Attitudes, Practices and Experiences*, Unpublished M.Sc. Dissertation, South Bank Polytechnic, London.

French, S. (1987), 'Attitudes of Physiotherapists to the Recruitment of Disabled and Handicapped People into the Physiotherapy Profession', *Physiotherapy*, Vol. 73, No. 7, pp. 363–367.
French, S. (1988), 'Experiences of Disabled Health and Caring Professionals', *Sociology of Health and Illness*, Vol. 10, No. 2, pp. 170–188.
French, S. (1990a), 'The Advantages of Visual Impairment – Some Physiotherapists Views', *New Beacon*, Vol. 74, No. 872, pp. 1–6.
French, S. (1990b), 'Visually Handicapped Physiotherapists: Are Their Educational Needs Being Met?', *Educare*, Vol. 37, pp. 12–17.
French, S. (1991), 'What's So Great About Independence?', *New Beacon*, Vol. 75, No. 886, pp. 153–156.
French, S. (1993a), 'Can You See the Rainbow?: The Roots of Denial', in J. Swain, V. Finkelstein, S. French and M. Oliver (eds), *Disabling Barriers – Enabling Environments*, Sage, London, pp. 69–77.
French, S. (1993b), 'The Origins of Physiotherapy as a Career for Blind and Visually Impaired People', *Physiotherapy*, Vol. 79, No. 11, pp. 779–780.
French, S. (1994a), 'Physiotherapists Talking', *New Beacon*, Vol. 78, No. 921, pp. 14–17.
French, S. (1994b), 'Equal Opportunities? – Yes Please', in L. Keith (ed), *Musn't Grumble: An Anthology of Writing by Disabled Women*, The Women's Press, London, pp. 154–160.
French, S. (1995), 'Visually Impaired Physiotherapists: Their Struggle for Acceptance and Survival', *Disability and Society*, Vol. 10, No. 1, pp. 3–20.
French, S. (1996), 'Out of Sight Out of Mind: The Experience and Effect of a Special Residential School', in J. Morris (ed), *Encounters with Strangers: Feminism and Disability*, The Women's Press, London, pp. 17–47.
French, S. (1997a), 'Defining Disability: Its Implications for Physiotherapy Practice', in S. French (ed), *Physiotherapy: A Psychosocial Approach* (2nd ed), Butterworth-Heinemann, Oxford, pp. 336–350.
French, S. (1997b), 'Ageism'. in S. French (ed), *Physiotherapy: A Psychosocial Approach* (2nd ed), Butterworth-Heinemann, Oxford, pp. 73–85.
French, S. (1997c), 'Dimensions of Disability and Impairment', in S. French (ed), *Physiotherapy: A Psychosocial Approach* (2nd ed), Butterworth-Heinemann, Oxford, pp. 229–243.
French, S. (1997d), 'The Attitudes of Health Professionals Towards Disabled people', in S. French (ed), *Physiotherapy: A Psychosocial Approach* (2nd ed), Butterworth-Heinemann, Oxford, pp. 86–99.
French, S. (1998),' Surviving the Institution: Working as a Visually Disabled Lecturer in Higher Education', in D. Malina and S. Maslin-Prothero (eds), *Surviving the Academy: Feminist Perspectives*, Palmer Press, London, pp. 31–41.
French, S. (2000), *Barriers and Coping Strategies: A Study of the Working Lives of Visually Impaired Physiotherapists*, Unpublished PhD thesis, Open University, Milton Keynes.
French, S., Gillman, M. and Swain, J. (1997), *Working with Visually Disabled People: Bridging Theory and Practice*, Venture Press, Birmingham.

French, S. and Swain, J. (1997), *From a Different Viewpoint: The Lives and Experiences of Visually Impaired People*, Royal National Institute for the Blind, London.

French, S. and Swain, J. (2000), 'Personal Perceptions on the Experience of Exclusion', in M. Moore (ed), *Insider Perspectives on Inclusion: Raising Voices, Raising Issues*, Philip Armstrong Publications, Sheffield, pp. 18–35.

Friend, B. (1996), 'Less Stress Campaign', *Physiotherapy Frontline*, Vol. 2, No. 3, p. 12.

Fry, E. (1986), *An Equal Chance for Disabled People*, The Spastics Society, London.

Gerber, D.A. (2000), 'Introduction: Finding Disabled Veterans in History', in D.A. Gerber (ed), *Disabled Veterans in History*, University of Michigan Press, Michigan.

Gething, L. (1993), 'Attitudes towards People with Disabilities of Physiotherapists and Members of the General Public', *Australian Journal of Physiotherapy*, Vol. 39, No. 4, pp. 291–296.

Giddens, A. (1989), *Sociology*, Polity Press, Cambridge.

Gleeson, B.J. (1997) 'Disability Studies: A Historical Materialist View', *Disability and Society*, Vol. 12, No. 2, pp. 1179–202.

Goffman, I. (1968), *Stigma: Notes on the Management of a Spoiled Identity*, Penguin Books, Harmondsworth.

Goffman, I. (1969), *The Presentation of Self in Everyday Life*, Penguin Books, Harmondsworth.

Gooding, C. (1994), 'Will Employers Pay for the Privilege?' *Disability Issues*, Vol. 15, p. 5.

Gooding, C. (1995), 'Employment and Disabled People: Equal Rights or Positive Action?' in G. Zarb (ed), *Removing Disabling Barriers*, Policy Studies Institute, London, pp. 64–76.

Gooding, C. (1996), *Blackstone's Guide to the Disability Discrimination Act 1995*, Blackstone Press, London.

'The Government's New Deal for Disabled People' (1998), *New Beacon*, Vol. 80, No. 962, pp. 20–21.

Graham, P., Jordan, A. and Lamb, B. (1990), *An Equal Chance or No Chance?* The Spastics Society, London.

Gray, P. (1988), 'CSP Policy of Equal Opportunity for Part-Timers', *Physiotherapy*, Vol. 75, No. 5, pp. 255–261.

Greenwood, R. and Johnson, V.A. (1987), 'Employer Perspectives on Workers with Disabilities', *Journal of Rehabilitation*, Vol. 53, No. 3, pp. 37–45.

Gross, R.D. (1987), *Psychology: The Science of Mind and Behaviour*, Edward Arnold, London.

Hahn, H. (1990), 'Can Disability be Beautiful?' in N. Nagler (ed), *Perspectives on Disability*, University of Southern California Press, Palo Alto, pp. 310–319.

Hahn, H. (1997), 'Advertising the Acceptable, Employable Image: Disability and Capitalism', in L.J. Davis (ed), *Disability Studies Reader*, Routledge, London, pp. 172–186.

Hales, G. (ed) (1996), *Beyond Disability: Towards an Enabling Society*, Sage, London.

Harris, C. (1991a), 'Blind PT School Faces the Axe', *Therapy Weekly*, Vol. 17, No. 35, p. 1.
Harris, C. (1991b), 'PT School Closure Would Leave Blind Students in the Lurch', *Therapy Weekly*, Vol. 17, No. 36, p. 2.
Hasler, F. (1993), 'Developments in the Disabled People's Movement', in J. Swain, V. Finkelstein, S. French and M. Oliver (eds), *Disabling Barriers – Enabling Environments*, Sage, London, pp. 285–292.
Hayward, S. (1996), *Applying Psychology in Organisations*, Hodder and Stoughton, London.
Heiser, B. (1995), 'The Nature and Causes of Transport Disability in Britain and How to Remove it', in G. Zarb (ed), *Removing Disabling Barriers*, Policy Studies Institute, London, pp. 49–63.
Henshaw's Blind Asylum (1895), Annual Report, Manchester.
Hermeston, R. (1998), 'Labour Shows Its Hand', *Disability Now*, April, p. 15.
Hevey, D. (1992), *The Creatures Time Forgot: Photography and Disability Imagery*, Routledge, London.
Hughes, B. and Paterson, K. (1997), 'The Social Model of Disability and the Disappearing Body: Towards a Sociology of Impairment', *Disability and Society*, Vol. 12, No. 3, pp. 225–240.
Hughes, G. (1998), 'A Suitable Case for Treatment? Constructions of Disability', in E. Saraga (ed), *Embodying the Social: Constructions of Difference*, Routledge, London, pp. 43–90.
Hugman, R. (1991), *Power in the Caring Professions*, Macmillan, London.
Humphries, S. and Gordon, P. (1992), *Out of Sight: The Experience of Disability 1900–1950*, Northcote House, Plymouth.
Hurst, A. (1996), 'Equal Opportunities and Access: Developments in Policy and Provision for Disabled Students 1990–1995', in F. Wolfendale and J. Corbett (eds), *Opening Doors: Learning Support in Higher Education*, Cassell, London, 129–144.
Jacobson, B., Smith, A. and Whitehead, M. (1991), *The Nation's Health: A Strategy for the 1990s*, King Edward's Hospital Fund for London, London.
Jenkins, J. (1957) 'Physiotherapy: The Biggest Professional Outlet for the Blind in Britain', *New Beacon*, Vol. 51, No. 482, pp. 76–79.
Johnson, L. and Moxon, E. (1998), 'In Whose Service? Technology, Care and Disabled People: The Case for a Disability Politics Perspective, *Disability and Society*, Vol. 13, No. 2, pp. 241–258.
Jolly, D. (2000), 'A Critical Evaluation of the Contradictions for Disabled Workers Arising from the Emergence of the Flexible Labour Market in Britain', *Disability and Society*, Vol. 15, No. 5, pp. 795–810.
Kettle, M. (1979), *Disabled People and Their Employment*, Association of Disabled Professionals, Banstead.
Kitchen, B., Shirlow, P. and Shuttleworth, I. (1998), On the Margins: Disabled People's Experiences of Employment in Donegal West Ireland, *Disability and Society*, Vol. 13, No. 5, pp. 785–801.
Kubler-Ross, E. (1969), *On Death and Dying*, Tavistock Publications, London.
Lazarus, R.S. and Folkman, S. (1984), *Stress, Appraisal and Coping*, Springer, New York.

Leary, E. (1969), The Association of Blind Chartered Physiotherapists, *The Physiotherapists' Quarterly*, Golden Jubilee Edition 1919–1969.
Leicester, M. and Lovett, T. (1997) Disability Voice: Educational Experiences and Disability, *Disability and Society*, Vol. 12, No.1, pp. 111–118.
Lewis, V. (1987), *Development and Handicap*, Basil Blackwell, Oxford.
Libman, G. (1983), 'Doctor Who Overcomes Deafness', *Synapse*, Vol. 4, No. 5, pp. 2–3.
Local Government Management Board (1991), *Ability Counts*, London.
Lonsdale, S. (1985), *Work and Equality*, Longman, London.
Lonsdale, S. (1990), *Women with Disabilities: The Experience of Physical Disability among Women*, Macmillan, London.
Lovelock, R., Powell, J. and Craggs, S. (1995), *Shared Territory: Assessing the Social Support Needs of Visually Impaired People*, Joseph Rowntree Foundation, York.
Lunt, N. and Thornton, P. (1994), 'Disability and Employment: Towards an Understanding of Discourse and Policy', *Disability and Society*, Vol. 9, No. 2, pp. 223–238.
Manpower Services Commission (1984), *Code of Good Practice on the Employment of Disabled People*, London.
Martin, J., Meltzer, H. and Elliot, D. (1988), *The Prevalence of Disability Among Adults*, OPCS Surveys of Disability in Great Britain, Report 1, HMSO Publications, London.
Mason, M. (1992), 'Internalised Oppression', in R. Rieser and M. Mason (eds), *Disability Equality in the Classroom: A Human Rights Issue* (2nd ed), Disability Equality in Education, London, pp. 27–28.
Maw, S. (1983), *The Provision of Post-Registration Courses for the Visually Handicapped Physiotherapist*, Diploma in Management Studies (Education), Unpublished Project, North East London Polytechnic, London.
McCall, S. (1994), 'Communication – Options and Issues', in D.T. Etheridge and H.L. Mason (eds), *The Visually Impaired: Curricula Access and Entitlement in Further Education*, David Fulton Publishers, London, pp. 96–109.
McConkey, R. and McCormack, B. (1983), *Breaking Barriers: Educating People about Disability*, Souvenir Press, London.
McDonald, P. (1996), 'A Disabled Student in Higher Education: Moving Beyond Segregation', in F. Wolfendale and J. Corbett (eds), *Opening Doors: Learning Support in Higher Education*, Cassell, London, pp. 117–128.
Mercer, J. (1978), *Aspects of Professionalisation in Physiotherapy, with some reference to other professions*, Unpublished Ph.D.Thesis, Institute of Education, London University.
Ministry of Labour and National Service (1951), *Report of the Working Party on the Employment of Blind Persons*, HMSO Publications, London.
Moon, P. (1990), *What Happens When Nurses Become Disabled?*, The Royal Association for Disability and Rehabilitation, London.
Morris, J. (1989), *Able Lives: Women's Experience of Paralysis*, The Women's Press, London.
Morris, J. (1991), *Pride Against Prejudice: Transforming Attitudes to Disability*, The Women's Press, London.

Morris, J. (ed) (1996), *Encounters with Strangers: Feminism and Disability*, The Women's Press, London.

Mottram, E. and Flin, R.H. (1988). 'Stress in Newly Qualified Physiotherapists', *Physiotherapy*, Vol. 74, No. 12, pp. 607–812.

Myers, L. and Parker, V. (1996), 'Extending the Role of the Co-ordinator for Disabled Students', in F. Wolfendale and J. Corbett (eds), *Opening Doors: Learning Support in Higher Education*, Cassell, London, pp. 66–83.

North London School of Physiotherapy for the Visually Handicapped (1981), *Promotional Literature*, London.

North London School of Physiotherapy for the Visually Handicapped (1990), *Physiotherapy with Human Sciences Curriculum*, London.

Ogden, J. (1996), *Health Psychology*, Open University Press, Buckingham.

Oliver, M. (1990), *The Politics of Disablement*, Macmillan, London.

Oliver, M. (1991), 'Disability and Participation in the Labour Market', in P. Brown and R. Scase (eds), *Poor Work*, Open University Press, Milton Keynes, pp. 132–145.

Oliver, M. (1993a), 'Re-defining Disability: A Challenge to Research,' in J. Swain, V. Finkelstein, S. French and M. Oliver (eds), *Disabling Barriers – Enabling Environments*, Sage, London, pp. 69–77.

Oliver, M. (1993b), 'Disability and Dependency: A Creation of Industrial Societies? in J. Swain, V. Finkelstein, S. French and M. Oliver (eds), *Disabling Barriers – Enabling Environments*, Sage, London, pp. 69–77.

Oliver, M. (1996a), 'A Sociology of Disability or a Disablist Sociology?' in L. Barton (ed), *Disability and Society: Emerging Issues and Insights*, Longman, London, pp. 18–42.

Oliver, M. (1996b), Understanding Disability: From Theory to Practice, Macmillan, London.

Oliver, M. (1996c), 'Defining Impairment and Disability: Issues at Stake', in C. Barnes and G. Mercer (eds), *Exploring the Divide: Illness and Disability*, The Disability Press, Leeds, pp. 39–54.

Oliver, M. and Barnes, C. (1998), *Disabled People and Social Policy*, Longman, London.

Oliver, M. and Sapey, B. (1999), *Social Work with Disabled People* (2nd ed), Macmillan, London.

Out of Sight – Out of Work? (1996), *New Beacon*, Vol. 80, No. 947, pp. 23–24.

Owen Hutchinson, J. (1994a), Physiotherapy: Career Opportunities for Visually Impaired People – 2, *New Beacon*, Vol. 78, No. 921, pp. 4–12.

Owen Hutchinson, J., Atkinson, K. and Orpwood, J. (1998), *Breaking Down Barriers: Access to Further and Higher Education for Visually Impaired Students*, Stanley Thornes, Cheltenham.

Parr, S., Byng, S. with Gilpin, S. (1997), *Talking About Aphasia: Living With Loss of Language After Stroke*, Open University Press, Buckingham.

Parrish, R.K. (1988), 'How Do We Deal with Our Own Feelings About Blindness?', *Archives of Ophthalmology*, Vol. 105, pp. 31–33.

Pfeiffer, D. and Yoshida, Y. (1995), 'Teaching Disability Studies in Canada and the USA', *Disability and Society*, Vol. 10, No. 4, pp. 475–500.

Physiotherapy (1994a), 'Continuing Professional Development: What is it and What Does it Mean?', Vol. 80, No. 9, p. 623.

Physiotherapy (1994b), 'A Century of Physiotherapy, Great Britain and the World', Vol. 80A, pp. 11A–19A.

Physiotherapy (1994c), 'Equal Opportunities in Employment', Vol. 80, No. 5, pp. 296–8.

Physiotherapy Frontline (1995), 'Members with Disabilities Network Group, Vol. 1, No. 18, p. 18.

Physiotherapy Frontline (1996), 'Dramatic Increase in Disability Network', Vol. 2, No. 2, p. 7.

Physiotherapy Frontline (1997a), 'Student News', Vol. 3, No. 23, p. 12.

Physiotherapy Frontline (1997b), 'Disability Needn't Become a Handicap', Vol. 3, No. 1, p. 9.

Physiotherapy Frontline (1997c), 'Network Involved in Reviewing Publications for Accessibility', Vol. 3, No. 6, p. 9.

Physiotherapy Frontline (1999), 'Compensation Battle Won by Physio', Vol. 5, No. 10, p. 16.

Pointon, A. and Davies, C. (1997), *Framed: Interrogating Disability in the Media*, British Film Institute, London.

Polgar, S. and Thomas, S.A. (1995), *Introduction to Research in the Health Sciences* (3rd ed), Churchill Livingstone, Edinburgh.

Porteous, M. (1997), *Occupational Psychology*, Prentice-Hall, London.

Potts, M. and Fido, R. (1991), '*A Fit Person to be Removed: Personal Accounts of Life in a Mental Deficiency Institution*', Northcote House, Plymouth.

Preece, J. (1995), 'Disability and Adult Education: The Consumer View', *Disability and Society*, Vol. 10, No. 1, pp. 87–102.

Preece, J. (1996), 'Class and Disability: Influences on Learning Expectations', *Disability and Society*, Vol. 11, No. 2, pp. 191–204.

Prescott-Clarke, P. (1990), *Employment and Handicap*, Social and Community Planning Research, London.

Priestley, M. (1999), *Disability Politics and Community Care*, Jessica Kingsley Publishers, London.

RADAR (1990), 'All Aboard? How Public Transport Caters for Disabled Passengers', *Contact*, Vol. 65, pp. 13–33.

RADAR (1993), *Disability and Discrimination in Employment*, London.

Roulstone, A. (1998), *Enabling Technology: Disabled People, Work and New Technology*, Open University Press, Buckingham.

Royal National Institute for the Blind (undated), *RNIB School of Physiotherapy 1915–1975*, London.

Royal National Institute for the Blind (1978), *Annual Report*, London.

Royal National Institute for the Blind (1995), *Blindness: The Daily Challenge*, London.

Royal National Institute for the Blind (1996a), *Employment: The Facts*, London.

Royal National Institute for the Blind (1996b), *Listening to Students: A Survey of the Views of Older Visually Impaired People*, London.

Royal National Institute for the Blind (1997), *Visually Impaired Students and the Workers' Educational Association: A Survey Report*, London.

Royal National Institute for the Blind (1998), *Within Reason: Access to Services for Blind and Partially Sighted People*, London.
Ryan, J. and Thomas, F. (1987), The Politics of Mental Handicap (2nd ed), Free Association Books, London.
Ryan, W. (1976), *Blaming the Victim*, Vintage Books, New York.
St. Dunstan's (undated), *An Ideal Occupation*, Public Relations Department, Brighton.
St. Dunstan's (1960), *War Blinded Physiotherapists at St. Dunstan's Conference*, Brief Report, Brighton.
St. Dunstan's Review (1970), The Ideal Profession, May, pp. 19–23.
Saraga, E. (1998), Abnormal, Unnatural and Immoral? The Social Construction of Sexualities, in E. Saraga (ed), *Embodying the Social: Constructions of Difference*, Routledge, London, pp. 139–188.
Scullion, P.A. (1999), 'Disability in a Nursing Curriculum', *Disability and Society*, Vol. 14, No. 4, pp. 539–599.
Seale, J.K. (1998), Two Perspectives on the Language of Special Needs Computing: Towards a Shared View, *Disability and Society*, Vol. 13, No. 2, pp. 259–267.
Shakespeare, T., Gillespie-Sells, K. and Davies, D. (1996), *The Sexual Politics of Disability*, Cassell, London.
Shearer, A. (1981), *Disability: Whose Handicap?*, Basil Blackwell, Oxford.
Simkiss, P., Garder, S. and Dryden, G. (1998), *What Next? The Experience of Transition: Visually Impaired Students, Their Education and Preparation for Employment*, Royal National Institute for the Blind, London.
Slack, S. (1998), 'I am More than my Wheels', in M. Corker and S. French (eds), *Disability Discourse*, Open University Press, Buckingham, pp. 28–37.
Sly, F. (1996) 'Disability and the Labour Market', *Labour Market Trends*, September, pp. 413–424.
Smith, B. (1996), 'Working Choices', in G. Hales (ed), *Beyond Disability: Towards an Enabling Environment*, Sage, London, pp. 145–150.
Stetten, D. (1983), 'Tomorrow's Physician', *Pharos*, Vol. 45, No. 3, pp. 35–41.
Stiker, H. (1999), *A History of Disability*, University of Michigan Press, Michigan.
Summerfield, P. (1996), 'The Women's Movement in Britain from the 1860s to the 1980s', in T. Coslett, A. Easton and P. Summerfield (eds), *Women, Power and Resistance: An Introduction to Women's Studies*, Open University Press, Buckingham, pp. 227–237.
Sutherland, A.T. (1981), *Disabled We Stand*, Souvenir Press, London.
Swain, J., Finkelstein, V., French, S. and Oliver, M. (eds) (1993), *Disabling Barriers – Enabling Environments*, Sage, London.
Swain, J. and French, S. (1998), 'Measuring up to Normality: The Foundations of Disabling Care, in A. Brechin, J. Katz, J. Walmsley and S. Peace (eds), *Care Matters: Concepts, Practice and Research*, Sage, London, pp. 82–95.
Swain, J. and French, S. (2000), 'Towards An Affirmation Model of Disability', *Disability and Society*, Vol. 15, No. 4, pp. 169–182.
Swain, J., Gillman, M. and French, S. (1998), *Confronting Disabling Barriers: Towards Making Organisations Accessible*, Venture Press, London.
Swain, J. and Lawrence, P. (1994), Learning about Disability: Changing Attitudes or Challenging Understanding? in S. French (ed), *On Equal Terms: Working With Disabled People*, Butterworth-Heinemann, Oxford. pp. 87–102.

Teager, D.P.G. (1987), 'The Visually Handicapped Physiotherapist – The British Experience', *International Disability Studies*, Vol. 8, pp. 134–143.

Teager, D.P.G. (1994), 'Blind Physiotherapists: The Struggle for Acceptance', *Physiotherapy*, Vol. 80, A, pp. 11A–19A.

Thomas, M.G. (1957), *The Royal National Institute for the Blind 1868–1956*, Royal National Institute for the Blind, London.

Thompson, N. (1997), *Anti-Discriminatory Practice* (2nd ed), Macmillan, London.

Thompson, N. (1998), *Promoting Equality*, Macmillan, London.

Thornton, E. (1994), '100 Years of Physiotherapy Education', Physiotherapy, Vol. 80A, pp. 11A–19A.

Tillsley, C. (1997), 'Gaining Access to Employment Opportunities', *British Journal of Visual Impairment*, Vol. 15, No. 2, pp. 67–71.

Trade Union Disability Alliance (1997), *Why the Disability Discrimination Act must be Repealed and Replaced with Civil Right for Disabled People*, London.

Turner, C. (1984), 'Who Cares?', *Occupational Health*, Vol. 36, No. 10, pp. 449–452.

Union of the Physically Impaired Against Segregation (1976), *Disability Challenge*, May, Vol. 1.

Wainapel, S.F. and Bernbaum, M. (1986), 'The Physician with Visual Impairment and Blindness', *Archives of Ophthalmology*, Vol. 104, pp. 498–502.

Walker, R., Tobin, M. and McKennel, A. (1992), *Blind and Partically Sighted Children in Britain: The RNIB Survey*, Volume 2, HMSO Publications, London.

Weiner, G. (1998), 'Here a Little, There a Little: Equal Opportunity Policies in Higher Education in the UK', *Studies in Higher Education*, Vol. 23, No. 3, pp. 321–335.

Wendell, S. (1996), *The Rejected Body: Feminist Philosophical Reflections on Disability*, Routledge, London.

West, P. (1989), 'Income, Work and Disability', in D.L. Patrick and H. Peach (eds), *Disablement in the Community*, Oxford University Press, London, pp. 140–157.

Winyard, S. (1996), *Blind in Britain: The Employment Challenge*, Royal National Institute for the Blind, London.

Wolfendale, F. and Corbett, J. (eds) (1996), *Opening Doors: Learning Support in Higher Education*, Cassell, London.

Wolfensberger, W. and Tullman, S. (1989), 'A Brief Outline of the Principle of Normalisation', in A. Brechin. and J. Walmsley (eds), *Making Connections: Reflecting on the Lives and Experiences of People With Learning Difficulties*, Hodder and Stoughton, London, pp. 210–218.

Woolley, M. (1993), 'Acquired Hearing Loss: Acquired Oppression, in J. Swain, V. Finkelstein, S. French and M. Oliver (eds), *Disabling Barriers – Enabling Environments*, Sage, London, pp. 78–84.

Yoshimoto, T. (1901), Massage by the Blind in Japan, *The Blind*, Vol. 16, pp. 292–293.

Zarb, G. (ed) (1995a), *Removing Disabling Barriers*, Policy Studies Institute, London.

Zarb, G. (1995b), 'Modelling the Social Model of Disability', *Critical Public Health*, Vol. 6, No. 2, pp. 21–29.

Index

Abberley, P. 20, 37
Abercrombie, N. 8
absenteeism 19
access, barriers to *see* barriers
Access to Work initiative 25, 27, 119, 123, 124–6, 143, 178
administration
  as barrier to employment 83, 122–3
  coping strategies 123–9
  increase in 145–6
age
  onset of visual impairment 68
  profile of physiotherapy profession 69–70
Ajken, I. 15
Alfred Eichholz Clinic 61
Allen, M. 39
Allen, T. 5
American Society of Handicapped Physicians 42
anxiety 101–3
Apter, D. 33
Argyle, M. 138
arts 9–10
Ash, A. 93, 100
Ashley, Jack 29
assertive coping strategies 106–7
assistants *see* colleagues
Association of Blind Asians 9
Association of Blind Certified Masseurs 57–8, 60–1
Association of Blind Chartered Physiotherapists (ABCP) 57, 95, 107
Association of Manipulative Physiotherapists 161
Association of Visually Impaired Chartered Physiotherapists (AVICP) 57, 107
Atkinson, D. 5
Atkinson, R. L. 104, 135

attitudinal barriers 11, 15
  employment 22–4, 37–42, 47–9, 139–40, 143
  physiotherapy education 46–7, 98–101
audiology work, attitudes towards recruitment of disabled colleagues 41
audiotape, availability of course material on 95
avoidance 104, 107

Balser, R. 19
Barclay, J. xi, 53, 55–6, 59
Barnes, C. xvi, 3, 5, 6, 7, 10, 12, 13, 19, 20, 21, 23, 24, 27, 89, 102, 108, 118, 123, 137, 140, 141
Barnes, H. xi, 17, 18, 20, 21, 22, 23, 24, 28, 33, 34, 35, 37, 117, 161, 172, 174, 177, 179
Baron, S. 21, 27, 28, 102, 105, 108
barriers
  employment 13, 21–4, 117–44
    administration 83, 122–9
    attitudinal 22–4, 37–42, 47–9, 139–40, 143
    behaviour of colleagues 139–40
    environmental 11, 129–37
    findings of study 170–3
    meetings 137–9
    narratives 157–65
    therapeutic equipment 120–2
    transport 21, 117–20
  in physiotherapy education 94–101, 113–14
  see also social model of disability
Bennet, G. 42
Bernbaum, M. 42
biopsychosocial model of disability 4
Birse, E. 39
Borland, J. 93, 98, 100

193

Bourke, J. 56
Bradfield, A. L. 21–2
braille 21, 95, 124
British Council of Disabled People (BCODP) 9
British Council of Organisations of Disabled People (BCODP) 9
British Deaf Association 8
British and Foreign Blind Association 53, 54, 55
British Society of Audiology 41
Broom, J. P. 127, 128, 174
Bruce, I. xiv, 32, 33, 67, 68, 77, 131
Burchardt, T. 17, 18, 20, 22, 26, 27, 33, 34, 37, 117, 119, 160, 179
Burnfield, A. 42

Campbell, J. 9, 21, 114
Casserley, C. 32
Chartered Society of Massage and Remedial Gymnastics 53
Chartered Society of Physiotherapy (CSP) xii, 136
  attitude to recruiting disabled people 37–8, 69, 72
  continuous professional development and xiii
  definition of physiotherapy xii
  Disability Network 140, 142, 148, 153
  discrimination and 40, 140, 148, 164
  history 53
  relationship with visually impaired physiotherapists xi, xv, 58–60, 72, 153–4, 155, 172
Chinnery, B. 23, 40
citizenship concept 13
City Clinic 57
Clarke, J. 18
class *see* social class
clients, help from 135–7
colleagues
  attitudes towards recruitment of disabled colleagues 37–42, 47–9
  behaviour as barrier to employment 139–40
  help from
    in employment 123–4, 128–9, 133–5, 139
    in physiotherapy education 105–6, 107–8
College of Radiographers 41
Colorez, A. 39
community work 77, 118, 119
compensation as coping strategy 108, 140, 141–2
computers 124–6
Cooper, J. 29
Cooper, N. 4
coping strategies
  employment
    administration 123–9
    compensation 108, 140, 141–2
    environmental barriers 133–7
    findings of study 173–4
    meetings 138–9
    minimisation 108, 140, 141
    narratives 157–65
    openness 108, 140, 142–3
    therapeutic equipment 121–2
    transport 119–20
  physiotherapy education 103–8, 114
    attending with sighted person 105–6
    avoidance and use of special courses 104, 107
    being proactive and assertive 106–7
    spontaneous help 107–8
Corbett, J. 29, 106
Corley, G. 5
Cornes, P. 25, 26
Council for Professions Supplementary to Medicine (CPSM) xii, 63
counsellors, experiences of disabled people as 44
courtesy stigma 38, 100
Craik, C. 42
Crow, L. xvi, 12, 114
Curtis, J. 33, 95, 98, 109

Davis, K. 8, 9, 40
deaf people 7

experiences as health and welfare professionals 43, 44–5, 46, 47, 48
Dench, S. 28, 33
Department of Employment, two tick symbol 24–5
dependency 24, 40, 137
Deshen, S. 24, 34
Disability Advisory Service 25
Disability Discrimination Act 1995 xv, 12, 17, 29–32, 37, 67, 92, 113, 126, 143, 146, 154, 155, 171, 177, 178, 179
Disability Network 140, 142, 148, 153
Disability Rights Commission 31
disability studies xv-xvi
disabled people and disability
  barriers for *see* barriers
  institutional discrimination 3, 12–15, 143
  models 3–15
    biopsychosocial model 4
    definition of model 3–4
    individual model xvi, 3, 4–7, 26
    medical model 4–5, 100
    religious model 3
    social model xvi, 3, 7–12
  perceptions and experiences of disabled health and welfare professionals 43–9
    access to professional education 45–6
    advantages and disadvantages of being disabled 43–5
    employment 47–9
    see also study of visually impaired people in physiotherapy
Disabled People's International (DPI) 9
disabled people's movement 3, 8–10
Disabled Persons Employment Act 1944 17, 24, 25
Disablement Income Group (DIG) 9
discrimination 40, 140, 148, 164
  institutional 3, 12–15, 143
  see also barriers
doctors, experiences of disabled people as 42, 44, 45, 46–7, 48

Dodds, A. G. 21
Downs, C. 123
Doyle, B. J. 29, 126
Duckett, P. S. 46, 147, 148
Dyer, L. 23

East London University 64
education 5, 13, 30, 32
  access to professional education 45–6
  in physiotherapy 72–6, 93–115
    attitudinal problems 46–7, 98–101
    barriers 94–101, 113–14
    coping strategies 103–8, 114
    feelings of embarrassment and anxiety 101–3
    post-registration 93–115
    views on integrated education 73–6, 108–13, 115
  social class and 71–2
Edwards, K. 39, 40
Eichholz, Alfred and William 61
electrotherapy 59–60, 121
Elliott, D. L. 39
embarrassment 101–3, 113
embodiment, culture of 4
emotion-based coping 104
employment 17–35
  barriers 13, 21–4, 117–44
    administration 83, 122–9
    attitudinal 22–4, 37–42, 47–9, 139–40, 143
    behaviour of colleagues 139–40
    environmental 11, 129–37
    findings of study 170–3
    meetings 137–9
    narratives 157–65
    therapeutic equipment 120–2
    transport 21, 117–20
  changing work environment 145–55
    impact of NHS and Community Care Act 1990 xv, 122, 144, 145–6, 155, 179
    job satisfaction 149–51
    promotion 146–9
    suitability of physiotherapy as career for visually impaired

people 152–5
comparison of visually impaired and
    sighted physiotherapists 76–84
findings of study 169–70
coping strategies
    administration 123–9
    compensation 108, 140, 141–2
    environmental barriers 133–7
    findings of study 173–4
    meetings 138–9
    minimisation 108, 140, 141
    narratives 157–65
    openness 108, 140, 142–3
    therapeutic equipment 121–2
    transport 119–20
equal opportunities 27–9, 37
government schemes and 11, 24–7
job satisfaction 79–82, 149–51
perceptions and experiences of
    disabled health and welfare
    professionals 47–9
social and psychological benefits of
    work 19–21
suitability of physiotherapy as career
    for visually impaired people
    89–91, 152–5
visually impaired people 18, 21, 27,
    32–4, 35
see also Disability Discrimination
    Act 1995
environmental barriers 11, 129–33
    coping strategies 133–7
epilepsy 46
equal opportunities 27–9, 37
equipment as barrier to employment
    120–2
erythemameter 60

Farish, M. 27, 28, 29
Fernando, S. 40
Fido, R. 5, 6
Finkelstein, V. xvi, 3, 4, 6, 11, 13, 40,
    41
Fishbein, M. 15
Fletcher Little, J. 54–5, 179
Flyn, R. H. 127
Foley, C. 25, 31

Folkman, S. 104
Fraser, Ian 60
French, S. xi, xiv, 4, 5, 6, 7, 23, 24,
    26, 27, 37, 39, 40, 41, 43, 58,
    70, 78, 79, 80, 93, 94, 95, 99,
    102, 111, 118, 123, 131, 136,
    137, 154, 161, 172, 174, 179
Friend, B. 128
Fry, E. 23, 174

Geist, E. O. 39
GEMMA 9
gender
    attitudes to massage and 59
    discrimination 40
    gender balance in physiotherapy 69,
        163–4
Gerber, D. A. 56–7
Gething, L. 40
Giddens, A. 8
Gleeson, B. J. xvi
Goffman, I. 6, 7, 19, 38, 41, 99, 100,
    108, 141, 174, 177
Gooding, C. 25, 29, 30
Gordon, P. 5, 18, 161
government employment schemes 11,
    24–7
    Access to Work initiative 25, 27,
        119, 123, 124–6, 143, 178
Graham, P. 20, 23–4
Gray, P. 59
Greenwood, R. 19, 24
grief, stages of 6
Gross, R. D. 103–4
gynaecological work 78

Hahn, H. 17, 18, 99, 161
Hales, G. 5
harassment 140
Harris, C. 64
Harvey, B. 19
Hasler, F. 9
Hayward, S. 127, 128, 129, 135, 146
health and welfare professionals 37–49
    attitudes towards recruitment of
        disabled colleagues 37–42, 47–9
    perceptions and experiences of

disabled health and welfare professionals 43–9
  access to professional education 45–6
  advantages and disadvantages of being disabled 43–5
  attitudes and behaviour of teachers 46–7
  employment 47–9
  see also physiotherapy
Heiser, B. 119
help
  from colleagues
    in employment 123–4, 128–9, 133–5, 139
    in physiotherapy education 105–6, 107–8
  from patients and clients 135–7
Henshaw's Blind Asylum 54
Hermeston, R. 27
Hevey, D. 11–12
home workers 19
hospitals
  environmental barriers 129–33
  intensive care units 87, 132–3, 134–5, 162
  out-patient work 130–1, 136
Hughes, B. 173
Hughes, G. 3, 4
Hugman, R. 40, 41
Human Rights Act 1998 31–2
Humphries, S. 5, 18, 161
Hurst, A. 28

impairment
  Disability Discrimination Act 1995 and 29
  distinguished from disability 10–11
  visually impaired people in physiotherapy 67–9
incomes 18
Incorporated Society of Trained Masseuses (ISTM) 53, 55, 58–9
individual model of disability xvi, 3, 4–7, 26
information, accessibility of 123
institutional discrimination 3, 12–15, 143
intensive care units 87, 132–3, 134–5, 162
internal oppression 6–7, 102, 114

Jacobson, B. 41
James, S. 93, 98, 100
Jenkins, J. 57, 60, 61
job satisfaction 79–82, 149–51
Johnson, L. 26
Johnson, V. A. 19, 24
Jolly, D. 24

Kettle, M. 19
Kitchen, B. xi, 134, 141
Kubler-Ross, E. 6

Lambeth Council 17
Lawrence, P. 11, 28
Lazarus, R. S. 104
learning disabilities 5, 10, 22
Leary, E. 57–8
Leicester, M. 93, 103
Lewis, V. 39
Liberation Network of Disabled People 9
Liberty 31
Libman, G. 40
Local Government Management Board 19, 28
London Institute of Massage by the Blind 54–5
London School of Massage 54
Lonsdale, S. 7, 20, 21
Lovelock, R. 68
Lovett, T. 93, 103
Lunt, N. 27

McCall, S. 21
McConkey, R. 97
McCormack, B. 97
McDonald, P. 93, 102, 142
Manpower Services Commission 24
Martin, J. 32
Mason, M. 102
massage xi, xii, 53, 59
Maw, S. 58

meals 101
medical model of disability 4–5, 100
meetings as barrier to employment 137–8
  coping strategies 138–9
mental handicap (learning disabilities) 5, 10, 22
mental illness 10, 20, 157–9, 160–1
Mercer, J. 59, 70, 71
minimisation as coping strategy 108, 140, 141
models of disability 3–15
  biopsychosocial model 4
  definition of model 3–4
  individual model xvi, 3, 4–7, 26
  medical 4–5, 100
  religious 3
  social model xvi, 3, 7–12
    origins of 10–12
Moon, P. 38
Morris, J. xvi, 5, 7, 11, 18, 21, 23, 114, 134, 154
Mottram, E. 127
Moxon, E. 26
Myers, L. 28–9, 93, 94

National Federation of the Blind 9
National Health Service 61–3
  state registration of physiotherapists 63–4
National Health Service and Community Care Act 1990 67, 92, 171
  impact on visually impaired people in physiotherapy xv, 122, 144, 145–6, 155, 179
National Institute of Massage by the Blind 55
National League of the Blind 8
neurology 100
New Deal for Disabled People 27
new social movements 8
non-verbal communication 137–8
North London School of Physiotherapy 38, 54, 69, 72, 111–12
  closure 64–5, 67, 108, 112–13, 114–15
nurses, attitudes towards recruitment of disabled colleagues 38, 39

obstetric work 78
occupational therapists
  attitudes towards recruitment of disabled colleagues 39, 42, 48
  experiences of disabled people as 45, 46, 47, 48
Ogden, J. 104
Oliver, M. xvi, 4, 5, 6, 7, 8, 9, 10, 11, 12, 13, 19, 20, 21, 26, 28, 31, 40, 102, 114, 170
openness as coping strategy 108, 140, 142–3
out-patient work 130–1, 136
Owen Hutchinson, Jane 64, 65, 93, 98, 101, 104, 105, 123

paediatric work 78, 99
paperwork *see* administration
Parker, V. 28–9, 93, 94
Parr, S. 123
Parrish, R. K. 42
part-time employment 19, 78, 79
paternalism 40
Paterson, K. 173
patients, help from 135–7
Pfeiffer, D. xvi
physiotherapy xii-xiii
  age profile 69–70
  attitudes towards recruitment of disabled colleagues 39
  continuous professional development xiii, 93
  as degree profession xii, 60, 64
  education in 72–6, 93–115
    attitudinal problems 46–7, 98–101
    barriers 94–101, 113–14
    coping strategies 103–8, 114
    feelings of embarrassment and anxiety 101–3
    post-registration 93–115
    views on integrated education 73–6, 108–13, 115
  experiences of disabled people in

44, 46, 47
grades of physiotherapist xiii
social class profile 70–2, 151
state registration 63–4
Placement, Assessment and
    Counselling Teams (PACT) 25
Polgar, S. 3
Porteous, M. 127, 128, 129, 133, 149, 151
Potts, M. 5, 6
Pratt, S. 25, 31
Preece, J. 40, 103, 107
Prescott-Clarke, P. 17, 20
Priestley, M. 3, 7, 9
proactive coping strategies 106–7
problem-focused coping 104
productivity 19
Professions Supplementary to
    Medicine Act 1960 xiii, 63
promotion 146–9
prosthetists, experiences of disabled
    people as 43–4, 45
psychiatrists, experiences of disabled
    people as 45

race 40
Race Relations Act 1976 29, 30
radiography profession, attitudes
    towards recruitment of disabled
    colleagues 41
readers 123–4
reading speed 21
religious models of disability 3
Rights Now Campaign 31
Roulstone, A. 18, 22, 23, 25, 26, 27, 122
Royal Association for Disability and
    Rehabilitation (RADAR) 17, 19, 23, 24, 118
Royal National Institute for the Blind
    (RNIB) 32, 33, 98, 100–1, 103, 106, 118, 123, 131, 160
    New Deal and 27
    origins and history 54
    schools 68
    training in physiotherapy xi, xv, 38, 55, 56, 60, 61, 65, 69, 72, 111

    see also North London School of
        Physiotherapy
Ryan, J. 5
Ryan, W. 5

St. Dunstan's 56, 57, 59
Sapey, B. 4, 5, 6, 7
Saraga, E. 11, 18
Scullion, P. A. 39
Seale, J. K. 26
SEAwall of Institutional
    Discrimination 13, 14, 143
segregation 5
self-employment 33–4, 77
Sex Discrimination Act 1975 29, 30
Shakespeare, T. xvi
Shearer, A. 17, 20, 21
Shields, Clive 60
Simkiss, P. xi, xiv, 18, 22, 23, 27, 32, 33, 75, 86, 93, 106, 110, 117, 125, 126, 131, 139, 141, 148, 151, 172, 179
Slack, S. 131
Sly, F. 34, 77
Smith, B. 22
social class 40–1
    profile of physiotherapy profession
        70–2, 151
social model of disability xvi, 3, 7–12
    origins of 10–12
social side of courses 101
social workers
    attitudes towards recruitment of
        disabled colleagues 37
    experiences of disabled people 44, 45, 47, 96, 108
Society of Remedial Gymnasts 59
Society of Trained Masseuses (STM) 53
Spastics Society (Scope) 23
Special Aids to Employment Scheme
    (SAE) 25
spontaneous help 107–8
status, occupational 18, 34
Stetten, D. 42
stigma 38, 99, 100
Stiker, H. 3

stress 127–8, 135, 146
structural barriers 11
Stuart, O. 6, 40, 41
study of visually impaired people in physiotherapy xi
　changing work environment 145–55
　　impact of NHS and Community Care Act 1990 xv, 122, 144, 145–6, 155, 179
　　job satisfaction 149–51
　　promotion 146–9
　　suitability of physiotherapy as career for visually impaired people 152–5
　comparison of visually impaired and sighted physiotherapists 67–92
　　attitudes to visually impaired physiotherapists 84–9
　　career posts 83–4
　　demographic details 69–70
　　details of impairment 67–9
　　education in physiotherapy 72
　　employment 76–84
　　findings of study 169–70
　　grades 82–3
　　job satisfaction 79–82
　　perceived suitability of physiotherapy as career for blind and partially sighted people 89–91
　　socioeconomic status 70–2
　　views on integrated pre-registration physiotherapy education 73–6
　conclusions 169–80
　education in physiotherapy 72–6, 93–115
　　barriers 94–101, 113–14
　　coping strategies 103–8
　　feelings of embarrassment and anxiety 101–3
　　views on integrated education 73–6, 108–13, 115
　field of study xv-xvi
　historical overview 53–65
　　Association of Blind Certified Masseurs 57–8
　　closure of North London School of Physiotherapy 64–5, 67
　　influence of world wars 55–7
　　National Health Service 61–3
　　recognition of visually impaired physiotherapists 60–1
　　relationship between visually impaired physiotherapists and the Chartered Society of Physiotherapy 58–60
　　state registration 63–4
　　training under Dr Fletcher Little 54–5
　insights from 174–7
　narratives 157–65
　outline of the study xiii-xiv, xvi-xviii
　rationale for study xiv-xv
　recommendations for practice and further research 177–8
　substantive findings 169–74
Summerfield, P. 8
Sutherland, A. T. 5, 7, 20, 24, 40, 41
Swain, J. 3, 5, 7, 11, 12, 13, 21, 28, 95, 98, 99, 118, 123, 131, 137, 143, 161, 170

teachers, attitudes and behaviour of 46–7
teaching
　speed of 96
　teaching aids 94–6
Teager, D. P. G. xiv, 42, 54, 59, 63–4
technology 25–7
　computers 124–6
temporary employment 19
therapeutic equipment as barrier to employment 120–2
Thomas, A. 5
Thomas, F. 5
Thomas, M. G. 53, 63
Thomas, S. A. 3
Thompson, N. 3, 6, 13, 18, 21, 27, 28, 98
Thornton, E. 53, 59
Thornton, P. 27
Tillsley, C. 33

time requirements of disabled people 21, 27, 96, 126–8
Trade Union Disability Alliance 29, 31
Trades Union Congress (TUC) 31
transport 30
  as barrier to education 97–8
  as barrier to employment 21, 117–19
    coping strategies 119–20
Tullman, S. 6–7
Turner, C. 42
turnover of staff 19
two tick symbol 24–5

ultra-violet light treatment 60
unemployment 17, 20, 33
Union of the Physically Impaired Against Segregation (UPIAS) 9, 10
United Nations 9
universities, physiotherapy as degree profession xii, 60, 64

venue, problems with 97, 98
Vernon, S. 29
victim blaming 5, 13
visual teaching aids 94–6
visually impaired people
  education and 5
  employment 18, 21, 27, 32–4, 35
  experiences as health and welfare professionals 44, 45, 46, 47
  physiotherapy and *see* study of visually impaired people in physiotherapy
reading speed 21

wages 18
Wainapel, S. F. 42
Walker, R. 33
Way, Percy 58, 59
Weiner, G. 70
welfare services *see* health and welfare professionals
Wendell, S. 5–6, 22, 23
West, P. 21
Whittington Hospital 61, 63
Williams, J. 127, 128, 174
Winyard, S. 33
Wolfendale, F. 106
Wolfensberger, W. 6–7
women
  gender discrimination 40
  women's movement 8
Woolley, M. 6, 7, 102

Yoshida, Y. xvi
Yoshimoto, T. 54

Zarb, G. 20, 21, 89, 98, 131, 177